Idiotypes and Lymphocytes

IMMUNOLOGY

An International Series of Monographs and Treatises

EDITED BY

F. J. DIXON, JR.
Division of Experimental Pathology
Scripps Clinic and Research Foundation
La Jolla, California

HENRY G. KUNKEL
The Rockefeller University
New York, New York

Idiotypes
and
Lymphocytes

CONSTANTIN A. BONA

Department of Microbiology
Mount Sinai School of Medicine
New York, New York

1981

ACADEMIC PRESS
A Subsidiary of Harcourt Brace Jovanovich, Publishers
New York   London   Toronto   Sydney   San Francisco

ACADEMIC PRESS, INC.
111 Fifth Avenue, New York, New York 10003

United Kingdom Edition published by
ACADEMIC PRESS, INC. (LONDON) LTD.
24/28 Oval Road, London NW1 7DX

Library of Congress Cataloging in Publication Data

Bona, Constantin.
    Idiotypes and lymphocytes.

    (Immunology; v. 6)
    Bibliography: p.
    1. Immunoglobulin idiotypes. 2. Lymphocytes.
I. Title. II. Series. [DNLM: 1. Immunoglobulin
idiotypes--Immunology. 2. B-Lymphocytes--Immunology.
3. T-Lymphocytes--Immunology. QW 575 B697i]
QR186.7.B66   616.07'9   81-10759
ISBN 0-12-112950-0   AACR2

PRINTED IN THE UNITED STATES OF AMERICA

81 82 83 84   9 8 7 6 5 4 3 2 1

To Henry Kunkel and Jacques Oudin
for their discovery of idiotypy

Contents

3 Variation of Idiotypes during the Immune Response

4 Expression of Idiotypes on B Cells

5 Idiotypic Determinants and T Cells

6 Immune Network: Regulation of Lymphocyte Functions by Anti-idiotype Antibodies

7 Physiological and Pathological Implications of the Immune Network

Preface

Idiotypy is one of the most innovative concepts in modern immunology, one which has constantly occupied the thoughts and labors of many immunologists for the past twenty years. After the discovery of antigenic individual specificities of human myeloma proteins, the concept of idiotypy applied to conventional antibodies has stimulated much research, with progress in several directions.

For several years, idiotypes were used as a tool to study the genetics and structure of antibodies and the mechanisms of generation of antibody diversity. After 1970, the idiotypic determinants as phenotypic markers of V region genes were used to identify the progeny of clones reactive to a particular antigen. These studies led to the conclusion that the same set of V genes encodes the specificity of the antigen-binding receptor of T and B lymphocytes. This concept opened the way for a new field of investigation focused on the physiological significance of idiotypes.

The discovery of autoanti-idiotype antibodies and of the antigen-mimicking properties of anti-idiotype antibodies, and that the idiotypic determinants borne by the lymphocyte's receptor serve as regulatory sites, led to the formulation of the network theory. This theory describes the immune system as a web of V domains in which the clones speak to one another using an idiotype dictionary. These numerous innovative concepts developed from the initial discovery of idiotypy are still to be applied to the physiology and pathology of lymphoid and nonlymphoid somatic cells. Therefore, we expect that the idiotypic tool will be used in coming years to broaden our understanding of the physiological host's defense immune reactions against viruses, bacteria, parasites, and tumor cells and that anti-idiotypic antibodies will be used to manipulate autoimmune diseases, age-related immune phenomena, and undesirable immune reactions such as graft rejection and hypersensitivity reactions.

The aims of this monograph are to present the progress made in the study of the idiotypes of lymphocytes and the various experimental findings demonstrating that a vast spectrum of possible relationships between cells and antibodies and communications between various subsets of T and B lymphocytes exist within the immune system.

The findings which led to the elucidation of the suppression-activation pathways of lymphocyte function as a result of the interaction of the receptors with the anti-idiotypic antibodies are of prime interest in the biomedical sciences. However, the complete elucidation of the complexity of the relationships and communications between cells and the physiological significance and pathological implications of the immune network require new investigations in which the immune functional network is dissected in detail.

We hope that the knowledge of the idiotypy of lymphocytes reviewed in this book will help the development of new directions in the research of the idiotypy of antibodies, particularly on the role of the idiotype–anti-idiotype reaction in various diseases. Our hopes are based on the simple concept that "new" ideas emerge from "old" observations and ideas.

I thank Monique and Alexandra for their help during the last two years while I prepared the manuscript of this monograph.

C. Bona

La nature a mis toutes ses verités chacune en soi-meme, notre art les renferme les unes dans les autres, mais cela n'est pas naturel: chacune tient sa place.

Blaise Pascal, *Pensées.*
Ed. 1678, chapitre **XXXI**, 21.

Idiotypy—General Features

I. Introduction

The majority of biological effectors of protein origin, such as hormones and enzymes, possess the ability to interact specifically with cell receptors or substrates, and they are immunogenic. Similarly, the antibody molecules, which represent the specific effectors of antibody-forming cells, exhibit a dual character; they interact specifically with antigens and are immunogenic by virtue of their protein nature as well as allotypic and idiotypic determinants.

The interaction with antigen is based on the extraordinary capacity of the immune apparatus to produce combining sites complementary to antigens. Recent estimates indicate that about 10^7 clones of antibody-forming cells synthesize an equal number of combining sites (Kabat, 1976). This extraordinary variability is contained in structural differences of combining sites of immunoglobulin (Ig) molecules which represent a segment of 5–34 Å. The combining site specificity as well as its three-dimensional structure is the result of noncovalent interactions between variable regions of the light and heavy chains of Ig molecules. In fact, the first structural study of two Bence-Jones myeloma proteins, which represent the light chain of Ig molecules (Hilschman and Craig, 1965), showed that the light chain can be divided into two regions: a variable region which differs in sequence from one Bence-Jones protein to another, and a constant region which shows a similar sequence. New structural and molecular findings clearly established that both heavy and light chains are composed of four segments: variable (V), diversity (D), joining (J), and constant (C). The genetic message of these regions is encoded by corresponding genes.

The variable region of both the heavy and light chains is constituted by three hypervariable and framework regions. The substitutions in hypervariable regions account for the extraordinary variety of combining sites of antibody molecules.

Immunogenicity of the antibody molecule is related to the antigenic determinants borne by both constant and variable regions of antibodies. Discovery of allotypy (Oudin, 1960) and localization of allotypic determinants in the constant regions (Koshland, 1967; Prahl and Porter, 1968) showed the immunogenic potency of antigenic determinants associated with the constant region of Ig molecules in homologous animals.

The discovery of idiotypy (Oudin and Michel, 1963; Kunkel et al., 1963) and the localization of idiotypic determinants in the variable regions (Grey et al., 1965; Wells et al., 1973) demonstrated the immunogenicity of antigenic determinants of the V region of Ig molecules.

The ensuing years have seen the accumulation of several important findings which show that idiotypic specificity is associated with a particular antigenic specificity of the antibody molecule. Resolution of this observation proved to be a crucial discovery, providing new insights about the diversity of antibodies and the regulation of the immune response.

Idiotypy is defined as the property of an antibody of expressing individual antigenic specificities both among antibodies of one individual against different antigens and among antibodies of several individuals against the same antigen. The individual antigenic specificities of Ig molecules were discovered by studying the immunogenicity of human myeloma proteins. Slater, Ward, and Kunkel in 1955 reported that rabbit antisera against one myeloma protein continued to react with this protein after extensive absorption of the antisera on normal Ig or other myeloma proteins. In 1963, Oudin and Michel in rabbits and Kunkel et al. (1963) in man showed that each antibody which interacted with a particular antigen expressed an individual antigenic specificity. This individual antigenic specificity of the antibody

molecule was called idiotype, a Greek name signifying individual form
or type, by Oudin and Michel (1969a).

II. Anti-idiotypic Sera

The idiotypes expressed on antibody molecules are defined roughly
by anti-idiotypic sera and more precisely by their structural correlates.
Anti-idiotypic sera can be obtained by immunization with antigen–
antibody complexes as Oudin and Michel (1963) prepared the anti-
idiotypic sera in rabbits, or with soluble, polymerized or carrier
coupled purified antibody or myeloma protein. Specificity of anti-
idiotypic sera obtained by these various methods of immunization is
very variable, since B cells which are able to make anti-idiotypic antibodies recognize many different idiotypes carried by the antibody
molecule. Thus, Jorgensen *et al.* (1977) studied the specificity of anti-
idiotypic antibodies produced by BALB/c mice after immunization
with MOPC315 myeloma protein, either alone or affinity labeled with
bromoacetyl-DNP-L-lysine. MOPC315 myeloma protein binds DNP
and TNP haptens. After immunization with MOPC315 myeloma protein alone, an anti-Id serum was obtained which reacted with idiotypic
determinants associated with the combining site, since the reaction
between MOPC315 and anti-Id antibodies was inhibited by DNP
ligands. In contrast, after immunization with MOPC315 affinity
labeled with bromoacetyl-DNP-L-lysine, the anti-Id antibodies found
were directed against idiotypes not associated with the combining site
since the binding of these antibodies to MOPC315 was not inhibited
by DNP-ligands. Similar results were obtained by Klaus (1978) after
immunization with a complex of KLH-DNP mixed in various ratios
with MOPC315. However, there is no general rule according to which
the antibody–antigen complex induces synthesis of anti-Id antibodies
against idiotypes associated with framework residues, and soluble or
polymerized antibodies are able to induce synthesis of anti-idiotypic
antibodies specific for idiotypes associated with the combining site.

Four categories of anti-idiotypic sera can be obtained as follows:

1. Heterologous anti-idiotypic sera obtained by immunization
across species barriers

2. Homologous anti-idiotypic sera obtained by immunization across
strain barriers

3. Syngeneic anti-idiotypic sera obtained by immunization in an inbred strain

4. Autologous anti-idiotypic sera obtained by immunization of the same individual (i.e., donor of antibody)

The heterologous and homologous anti-idiotypic sera are relatively easy to obtain; however, the induction of syngeneic and autologous anti-Id sera requires particular methods of immunization such as polymerization of purified antibodies or their coupling to heterologous protein carriers (Urbain, 1977; Rodkey, 1974; Bona *et al.*, 1979a).

The preparation of syngeneic anti-idiotypic sera by immunization with myeloma proteins depends on the sharing of idiotypic determinants borne by myeloma protein with "natural" antibodies elicited by environmental antigens.

In this context myeloma proteins can be classified into two categories:

a. Myeloma proteins which express idiotypes which do not exist in the serum of normal animals. In this case, anti-Id antibodies can be easily prepared in the syngeneic system as was shown by Sakato and Eisen (1975) for MOPC460, MOPC315, MOPC167, etc., myeloma proteins. Syngeneic anti-Id antibodies were obtained by immunization with these myeloma proteins emulsified in Freund's complete adjuvant (FCA).

b. Myeloma proteins which share Id determinants with "natural" antibodies present in a significant titer in normal mice such as anti-levan, anti-inulin, anti-galactan, anti-phosphocholine and anti-$\alpha(1\rightarrow3)$ dextran antibodies. In these cases, anti-Id antibodies against EPC109-inulin binding, XRPC-24 galactan-binding, TEPC15-phosphocholine binding, and J558-$\alpha(1\rightarrow3)$ dextran-binding myeloma proteins cannot be induced in syngeneic BALB/c mice by simple immunization with myeloma proteins emulsified in FCA. However, syngeneic anti-Id antibodies were prepared against these myeloma proteins using new methods of immunization. Thus, anti-T15 Id antibodies have been prepared in BALB/c mice idiotype suppressed in neonatal life (Cosenza *et al.*, 1977). Syngeneic anti-J558 antibodies were prepared in BALB/c mice preimmunized with DNP–hen ovalbumin and challenged with DNP–J558 (Schuler *et al.*, 1977). Seppälä and Eichmann (1979) prepared a syngeneic antiserum against S117-*Streptococcus* A-binding myeloma protein which reacted only with "minor" Id determinants of this protein. We succeeded in preparing syngeneic anti-Id antibodies by immunization with KLH-affinity chromatography purified antibody conjugates (Bona *et al.,* 1979a).

The magnitude of antibody response elicited across species, strain, and syngeneic barriers is very similar. Schiff *et al.* (1979) compared the titer of anti-MOPC173 idiotype antibodies made in rabbit, A/J, and BALB/c mice. MOPC173 is a myeloma protein of BALB/c origin. Hemagglutination titer of rabbit anti-173 Id serum was 4×10^{-4}, of A/J mice 5×10^{-3} to 3×10^{-5}, and of BALB/c mice 2.5×10^{-3} to 1.6×10^{-4}.

III. Individual and Cross-Reactive Idiotypes

The idiotypy phenomenon was discovered in rabbits and humans, which are outbred species. Thus, for a long time it was considered that one antibody with a particular antigenic specificity produced by one individual expresses an idiotype which differs from any other individual. Accordingly, each antibody molecule could express only one idiotypic specificity, a "private" or "individual idiotype" (IdI).

Discovery of myeloma and Waldenstrom macroglobulins in humans and of myeloma proteins in mice (Potter and Boyce, 1962) gave new insight and a new tool to approach the study of idiotypy. Therefore, it was not until functionally related normal antibodies and myeloma proteins were studied that the cross-reactive idiotypes were identified (Kunkel *et al.,* 1973). Indeed, it was shown that antibodies induced by the same antigen in different individuals of an inbred strain, as well as myeloma proteins specific for the same hapten, can share a "common," "public," or cross-reactive idiotype (IdX). Serological and structural data clearly show that an antibody molecule of myeloma protein can express an IdI and an IdX. During the last few years, IdXs were identified on antibody molecules of outbred species. Williams *et al.* (1969) showed that some human myeloma proteins with anti-I agglutinin specificity shared an IdX. In the rabbit, which is an outbred species, common idiotypes were observed among the progeny of the same litter immunized with *Streptococcus* A (Eichmann and Kindt, 1974). Recently, Brandt and Jaton (1978) prepared in guinea pigs an anti-Id serum specific for a rabbit anti-pneumococcal type II polysaccharide antibody. This anti-idiotypic serum reacted with anti-pneumococcal antibodies of two rabbits among 30 rabbits studied.

The antibodies expressing the same idiotype from these two rabbits exhibited two antibody components with an indistinguishable isoelectric focusing pattern and a high degree of structural similarity. Aasted *et al.* (1976) have found a high degree of similarity among rabbit anti a series allotype antibodies with respect to L-chain binding patterns and major amino-terminal sequences.

IdXs can be classified in three major categories, which are presented below.

A. IdX Linked to Allotype

In some antibody responses developed by inbred mouse strains, the expression of IdX is controlled by genes linked to *Igh-C* genes. These IdXs are found in the strains which bear the same allotype. Examples of *V*-region IdX's controlled by *Igh-C* genes are provided in Section VII on the genetics of idiotypy.

The expression of Id determinants on the receptor of T cells is also linked to Igh-C genes (Binz and Wigzell, 1978; Bona and Paul, 1979b).

Structural data, as well as the inheritance of IdX in a Mendelian fashion, strongly suggest that IdX are products of germ line genes. In contrast, IdI, expressed on a unique myeloma protein or antibody produced by one individual of a strain of species which is not inherited, appears more consistent with a somatic mutation. Somatic mutations in immunological systems continue to represent an important mechanism of antibody diversity (Lederberg, 1973; Cohn, 1971).

B. Interstrain IdX

In contrast with IdXs linked to allotype, in other antigenic systems the *V*-region idiotypic determinants are expressed independently of the allotype carried by the antibody molecule.

Thus, the IdX of galactan-binding myeloma proteins was found on antigalactan antibodies produced by mice bearing Igh-C^a or -C^b allotypes (Mushinsky and Potter, 1977). Similarly, the GA-1 idiotype, which is expressed on a minor population of anti-GAT antibodies specific for "GA" immunodeterminants, was found in 18 mouse strains studied (Ju *et al.,* 1979b). This idiotype was identified using a homogenous anti-GAT antibody which lacked the major cGAT IdX borne by anti-GAT antibodies directed against the "GT" antigenic moiety of GAT polymer. The GA-1 idiotype was found on anti-GA antibodies produced in response to immunization with other GAT and also on anti-GA antibodies produced by immunization with other GA containing polymers such as GLA[40], GAT[33].

The 4.6 Id of monoclonal anti-SIII antibodies appears to be an interstrain IdX, since the guinea pig anti-Id sera raised against monoclonal 4.6 anti-SIII BALB/c antibodies interacted with anti-SIII antibodies produced by five mouse strains. Therefore, the expression of these interstrain IdXs is independent of *H-2* and *Igh-C* genes.

IdX on homologous anti-Ig antibodies represent another example of interstrain IdX. Such interesting IdXs were described in three systems.

1. IdX on Anti-IgG Antibodies

These were observed by Kunkel *et al.* (1973) on human monoclonal IgM proteins specific for human IgG (rheumatoid factor). The light chains of these proteins demonstrate a striking restriction of the V_L region subgroup (Capra *et al.*, 1973).

2. IdX on Anti-allotype Antibodies

We have recently shown (Bona, 1980b) that an idiotype expressed on BALB/c anti-IgG$_{2a}^b$ allotype antibodies produced by a single mouse was found on anti-allotype antibodies produced by all BALB/c mice as well as on anti-allotype antibodies produced by various responder strains of mice immunized with the CBPC 101 myeloma protein (Table 1.1). This myeloma protein is an IgG$_{2a}$ of CB20 mice origin which bears *Ig-1*^{b} allotype. This IdX was identified with BAB14 CxB1 and BC8 anti-Id antibodies which interact with BALB/c, BALB/B, C.AL20, P/J, and DBA/2 anti-IgG$_2$^{b} allotype antibodies (Table 1.2).

An IdX was found on anti-IgA^a allotype antibodies. We have raised in DBA/1 and DBA/2 mice anti Id antibodies against DBA/2 anti IgA^a allotype monoclonal antibodies. In B10 and CB20 mice we prepared an anti-Id antibody against a C.B20 anti-IgA^a monoclonal antibody.

These anti-Id antibodies agglutinated the SRBC coated with DBA/2 or CB20 anti-IgA^a allotype monoclonal antibodies (Table 1.3). Furthermore, this agglutination was inhibited by anti-IgA^a allotype antibodies produced by various strains of mice (Table 1.4). In rabbit it was also reported that anti-b4 and anti-a2 allotype antibodies bear a cross-reactive idiotype (Roland and Cazenave, 1979; Gilman-Sachs *et al.*, 1980).

TABLE 1.1

Expression of IdX(s) on Anti-Allotypes Antibodies Produced in Various Strains of Mice[a]

Strain immunized			Anti-(BALB/c anti-CBPC101)[b] produced in		Inhibition of binding of ^{3}H-labeled BALB/c anti-CBPC101 by BAB.14 anti-(BALB/c, anti-CBPC101)
	MHC type	Igh-C type	B.C8	BAB.14	
BALB/c	d	a	>8[c]	>8	1000[d]
BALB.B	b	a	3	6	10
B.C8	b	a	2	3	5
CXBG	b	a	4	6	30
CXBJ	b	a	3	4	3
129/SV	b	a	3	4	100
DBA/2	d	c	6	>8	1000
DBA/1	q	c	>8	5	100
C.AL20	d	a	7	>8	1000
RIII	r	g	6	>8	650
P/J	p	h	2	>8	650
SJA	s	a	>8	>8	1000

[a] From Bona et al., 1980b.

[b] Hemagglutination inhibition. SRBC coated with BALB/c anti-CBPC101.

[c] Reciprocal of the natural logarithm of the highest dilution causing inhibition of hemagglutination.

[d] Microtiter plates were coated with a 1 : 50,000 dilution of BAB.14 anti-(BALB/c anti-CBPC101) antiserum and incubated with 1 : 3, 1 : 10, 1 : 30, 1 : 100, 1 : 300, 1 : 1000, and 1 : 3000 dilutions of anti-allotype serum from various strains. In some experiments, other dilutions of inhibitors were used. ^{3}H-Labeled BALB/c anti-CBPC101 was used for binding. The result reported is the reciprocal of the highest dilution of anti-allotype serum causing more than 50% inhibition of binding.

3. IdX on Anti-Id Antibodies

BALB/c mice immunized with ABPC48 myeloma proteins develop a vigorous anti-A48Id antibody response. From these mice we obtained 17 hybridomas which secreted anti A48Id monoclonal antibodies. The binding of 16 anti-A48Id monoclonal antibodies to ABPC48 myeloma proteins was inhibited by bacterial levan. ABPC48 is an IgAk myeloma protein which binds $\beta(2\rightarrow6)$fructosan. We raised in BALB/c mice and W76 wild mice (bearing Igl[a] allotype) anti-Id

TABLE 1.2

Expression of IdX(s) on BALB/c, C.AL20, P/J, and DBA/2 Anti-Allotype
(IgG_{2a}^b) Antibody[a]

Strain in which anti-Id antiserum was produced	Immunogen Anti-CBPC101 produced in	HA titer (ln); SRBC coated with anti-CBPC101 antibody from			
		BALB/c	C.AL20	P/J	DBA/2
BAB.14	BALB/c	8	>8	>8	>8
CXBI	BALB/c	8	>8	>8	>8
B.C8	BALB/c	7	6	6	6
B.C8	BALB.B	7	6	8	8
B.C8	C.AL20	6	6	6	1
B.C8	P/J	5	0	5	5
B.C8	DBA/2	6	6	6	8

[a] From Bona *et al.,* 1980b.

antibodies against two anti-A48Id monoclonal antibodies (i.e., IDA3
and IDA10). These anti-Id antibodies reacted with ten anti-48Id
monoclonal antibodies as well as with heterogenous anti-A48Id antibodies produced by BAB.14 (Ig-1[b]), C.B20 (Ig-1[b]), and BALB/c
(Ig-1[a]) strains of mice (Table 1.5).

These data indicate than an interstrain IdX is expressed by
homologous anti-IgG, anti-allotype, and anti-Id antibodies which are

TABLE 1.3

Hemagglutination Titer of Monoclonal and Heterogenous Anti-Allotype
Antibodies Obtained from Various Strains of Mice Immunized with ABPC 48
(IgA[a]) Myeloma Protein

Origin of anti-allotype antibodies	HA titer (ln units)	
	ABPC-48-SRBC	MOPC384-SRBC
DBA/2 anti-IgA[a] monoclonal antibodies [F6(s)4]	27	25
C.B20 anti-IgA[a] monoclonal antibodies (EAall)	6	5
A/J anti-A48	12	7
C.B20 anti-A48	5	4
BALB/c anti-A48	6	0

TABLE 1.4

Hemagglutination Inhibition Tier of IdX Expressed on Anti-IgA^a Allotype Antibodies[a,b]

anti-ID sera	SRBC coated with monoclonal anti-IgA^a allotype antibodies	HI titer (ln)				
		EAall (1 mg/ml)	F6(5)4 (1 mg/ml)	A/He anti-IgA^a	A.L/N anti-IgA^a	C.B20 anti-IgA^a
DBA/1 anti-F$_6$(5)$_4$	F$_1$(5)$_4$	0	>8	0	4	0
DBA/1 anti-F$_6$(5)$_4$	EAall	>8	>8	ND^c	ND	ND
DBA/2 anti-F$_6$(5)$_4$	F$_6$(5)$_4$	>8	>8	4	3	0
DBA/2 anti-F$_6$(5)$_4$	EAall	>8	>8	ND	ND	ND
C.B20 anti-EAall	F$_6$(5)$_4$	0	>8	ND	ND	ND
C.B20 anti-EAall	EAall	>8	6	3	0	8
B10 anti-EAall	F$_6$(5)$_4$	3	>8	ND	ND	ND
B10 anti-EAall	EAall	>12	10	0	0	2

[a] These results were obtained in collaboration with P. A. Cazenave during my sojourn in the Department of Analytic Immunochemistry, Pasteur Institute, Paris.

[b] F$_6$(5)$_4$ are DBA/2 monoclonal anti-IgA^a antibodies; EAall are C.B20 anti-IgA^a antibodies. A/He anti-IgA^a allotype antibodies were obtained after subsequent immunization with TEPC803, A.L/N anti-IgA^a antibodies were obtained after immunization with HOPC 8, and C.B20 anti-IgA^a antibodies were obtained after immunization with ABPC48. TEPC803, HOPC8, and ABPC48 are IgA$_k^a$.

[c] ND, not done.

TABLE 1.5

IdX on Anti-48Id Antibodies[a]

	HI titer (ln)[b]		
Inhibitors	antiIDA$_3$ + IDA$_3$-SRBC	antiIDA$_3$ + IDA$_{10}$-SRBC	AntiIDA$_{10}$ + IDA$_3$-SRBC
Hybridoma (10 mg/ml)No.			
IDA$_3$	>12	4	4
IDA$_{15}$	0	3	4
IDA$_{10}$	0	5	4
IDA$_{14}$	0	2	3
IDA9	0	2	3
IDA6	11	2	2
IDA19	0	3	4
IDA13	0	0	4
IDA8	0	3	2
IDA5	0	3	3
IDA7	0	3	4
Anti-A48Id serum			
BALB/c	0	7	>8
C.B20	0	3	3
A/He	0	4	4
A/J	0	5	4
Anti-X24 serum			
C.B20	0	0	0
A/He	0	0	0

[a] These results were obtained in collaboration with P. A. Cazenave during my sojourn in the Department of Analytic Immunochemistry, Pasteur Institute, Paris.

[b] SRBC were coated with specifically purified monoclonal anti-48Id antibodies originating from BALB/c bearing IDA$_3$ and IDA$_{10}$ ascites.

independent of the *H-2 IgC* genes or other genetic markers. Furthermore, these data demonatrate that a single *V* gene or a very close family of germinal *V* genes which encode this homologous anti-Ig response was highly conserved during phylogeny. One may ask why the capacity to produce antibodies against antigenic determinants (i.e., allotype and idiotypes) borne by Ig molecules should be of such evolutionary significance that this ability would exhibit the degree of conservation observed. One obvious explanation that we have proposed (Bona, 1980b) is that *V* region genes which encode the combining portion of the H chain may also code for important molecules which normally regulate the expression of Ig classes. An alternative explanation is that the concentration of Ig represents an important parameter of any functional macromolecular homeostasis mechanism, and its maintenance within narrow limits requires conservation of this function during evolution.

C. Interspecies IdX

The presence of common idiotypic determinants on antibodies with the same antigenic binding activity produced by different animal species has also been identified.

1. ValIdX

Various animal species can make antibodies distinguishing between human adult hemoglobin and human sickle cell hemoglobin, which differ by one valine amino acid sutstitution called Val. Karol *et al.* (1977) prepared anti-Val antibodies in sheep, goat, and guinea pig immunized with sickle cell human hemoglobin. Anti-idiotypic antibodies were raised in rabbits. A strong cross-reactivity was observed between goat and sheep anti-Val antibodies, while guinea pig anti-Val antibody did not show cross-reactivity with sheep or goat anti-Val antibodies. These results indicate the existence of IdX on the antibodies produced by two closely related species.

2. cGATIdX

Idiotype analysis of antibodies to GAT showed them specific for "GT" immunogenic determinants. The IdX of anti-GAT antibody produced by one individual D1.LP mouse, used as immunogen to raise anti-Id antisera in the guinea pig, was shared by anti-GAT antibodies produced by various mouse strains as well as by several monoclonal anti GAT antibodies (Ju *et al.*, 1978a). The expression of cGATIdX in various strains of mice was independent of the expression of Ig-1, H-2 and V_K genetic markers. Furthermore, the cGATIdX was shared by rat (Ju *et al.*, 1978b) and guinea pig (Somme *et al.*, 1979) anti-GAT antibodies.

3. T15-IdX

IdX of TEPC15, HOPC8, and S107-phosphocholine-binding myeloma proteins were found on anti-phosphocholine antibodies produced in mice bearing Ig-1[a] allotype (Lieberman *et al.*, 1974). Recent data have shown that while the BALB/c Ig-1[a] allotype was closely related to the expression of T15-IdX on the humoral antibodies, it did not play a role at the precursor cell level. Cancro *et al.* (1978) have reported that RI CxB inbred strains and C.B20 mice which bear Ig1^b allotype expressed the T15-IdX at the precursor cell level. This suggests a regulation during or before antigenic stimulation rather than a specific clone expression in the antibody repertoire. Claflin and Davie (1974) found that one out of eight hamsters studied has produced T15-IdX anti-PC antibody. Interestingly, Riesen (1979) found a certain idiotypic similarity between a phosphocholine-binding human myeloma protein and murine MOPC603 myeloma protein which is also specific for this hapten.

The existence of interspecies IdX suggest that germ line genes coding for the variable region of antibodies may have evolved along with other genes in various mammalian species. The discovery of such IdX can represent a powerful taxonomic tool to unravel the evolutionary process and the relationship between species. The conservation during evolution of V_H structures encoding Val, T15, and cGAT idiotypes may indicate a selective advantage of these idiotypes for mammalian species.

IV. Triple Relationship between Combining Site, Hypervariable Region, and Idiotypes

Soon after the discovery of idiotypy of antibodies, the structures responsible for idiotypic specificity were located on Fab fragments (Grey *et al.*, 1965) and later on Fv fragments (Wells *et al.*, 1973) of Ig molecules. The variable region of a myeloma protein as well as any antibody molecule is constituted of three hypervariable regions and four framework segments. The framework segments of the light chain correspond to positions $1-23$ (Fr I), $35-43$ (FR 2), $57-88$ (FR 3), and 98–107 which is also considered J segment. Similarly, heavy chain framework segments correspond to 1–30, 36–44, 69–84, and 107–113 (Kabat *et al.*, 1979).

The relationship between the combining site and hypervariable regions has been proved by affinity labeling. Indeed, labeled DNP was specifically bound to the hypervariable region of DNP-binding MOPC315 myeloma protein (Haimovich *et al.*, 1972) and anti-DNP antibodies produced by guinea pig strain 13 (Ray and Cebra, 1972).

The relationship between combining site and idiotypes was studied by the inhibition by haptens of anti-idiotype/idiotype reactions. In these experiments, the binding of antigen to the combining site complementary structure of antibody molecules competed with the ability of anti-Id antibody to be bound to Id determinants. Inhibition of the anti-idiotype–idiotype reaction by haptens was observed in several systems, such as phenylarsonate antibody (Brent and Nisonoff, 1970) and anti A-CHO streptococcal antibodies (Briles and Krause, 1974). We showed that the Fc fragment of CBPC101 myeloma protein, which is an IgG_{2a}^b, inhibited the reaction between anti-Id antibodies directed against an IdX shared by anti-IgG_{2a}^b allotype antibodies produced by various strains of mice (Table 1.6).

Similarly, the binding of anti-Id antibodies to Id determinants of myeloma protein specific for $\alpha(1{\to}3)$dextran (Carson and Weigert, 1973), phosphocholine (Sher and Cohn, 1972), $\beta(2{\to}1)$fructosan (Lieberman *et al.*, 1975), $\beta(1{\to}6)$D-galactan (Potter *et al.*, 1973), and DNP and TNP (Sirisina and Eisen, 1971) was inhibited by corresponding haptens. However, it should be stressed that other Id determinants are not associated with the combining site since they are located in the framework segments. The existence of these two families of Id determinants, one associated with the combining site and the other with framework residues, was clearly demonstrated in several systems. Mudgett *et al.* (1978) prepared eight anti-Id sera against homogenous antibodies specific for *Streptococcus* C polysaccharide. The hapten of this particular polysaccharide is 3-O-2-N-acetylgalactosaminosyl-N-acetylgalactosamine. Some of these anti-Id sera contained a family of antibodies eluted by hapten, and a second population which was eluted by ammonium thiocynate. The hapten inhibitable reaction between anti-Id antibodies and idiotype was observed only in the case of antibodies eluted by hapten. Helman *et al.* (1976) prepared heterologous (rabbit) and syngeneic (BALB/c) anti-idiotypic antisera following immunization with Fv fragment of MOPC315 myeloma protein which is of BALB/c origin. They have found that rabbit anti-Id serum was predominantly (over 30%) anti-nonbinding site, whereas the syngeneic anti-Id serum was 60–70% inhibited by DNP hapten. An opposite situation was observed in the case of TEPC15-HOPC8 Id system in which the anti-T15IdX serum raised in rabbits reacted with combining site associated idiotypes whereas A/J anti-T15IdX interacts with framework associated IdX (Claflin and Davie, 1975). These findings show that we can distinguish two kinds of Id determinants: one associated with the combining site

TABLE 1.6

Inhibition of Binding of ^{3}H-Labeled Anti-CBPC101 Antibody to B.C8 and BAB.14 Anti-Id Sera by Fc Fragments of CBPC101 Myeloma Protein[a]

| | Anti-CBPC101 antibody; (% inhibition of binding in radioimmunoassay) | | | | | | | |
| | Plates coated with B.C8 anti-Id serum | | | | Plates coated with BAB.14 anti-(BALB/c anti-CBPC101) | | | |
Inhibitors	^{3}H-labeled BALB/c[b]	^{3}H-labeled C.AL20[c]	^{3}H-labeled P/J[d]	^{3}H-labeled DBA/2[e]	^{3}H-labeled BALB/c	^{3}H-labeled C.AL20	^{3}H-labeled P/J	^{3}H-labeled DBA/
BALB/c anti-CBPC101 (1 mg/ml)	97	—	—	—	96	—	—	—
C.AL20 anti-CBPC101 (1.3 mg/ml)	—	85	—	—	—	95	—	—
P/J anti-CBPC101 (1 mg/ml)	—	—	89	—	—	—	93	—
DBA/2 anti-CBPC101 (0.4 mg/ml)	—	—	—	52	—	—	—	81
Fc fragment of CBPC101 (75 µg/ml)	98	95	97	96	98	88	95	94
UPC10 (10 mg/ml)	3	5	18	4	2	11	6	4

[a] From Bona et al., 1980b.
[b] Plates coated with B.C8 anti-(BALB/c anti-CBPC101).
[c] Plates coated with B.C8 anti-(C.AL20 anti-CBPC101).
[d] Plates coated with B.C8 anti-(P/J anti-CBPC101).
[e] Plates coated with B.C8 anti-(DBA/2 anti-CBPC101).

which is hapten inhibitable and another associated with the framework segments which is not inhibitable by haptens.

However, it should be stressed that the losing of the ability of antibody to interact with anti-idiotypes following combination with antigen does not necessarily indicate that idiotypes are associated with the combining site. In a striking example Kunkel *et al.* (1976) showed that Fab fragment of anti-Rh antibodies bound to red cells lost the reactivity of its idiotypic and subgroup related antigenic determinants. The binding with a large antigen such as the erythrocytes can profoundly alter the exposure of various antigenic determinants.

The relationship between hypervariable regions and idiotypes has also been proved by structural studies. Capra and Kehoe (1974) have performed the complete analysis of heavy and light chain variable regions of two human IgM myeloma proteins with anti-IgG activity which expressed an IdX. They found only eight amino acid differences in the entire variable region of their heavy chains, and three of them were in the hypervariable region. Study of the complete light chain sequence of IdX bearing anti-phenylarsonate antibodies produced in A/J mice indicated that all three hypervariable regions of three light chains exhibited a homogeneous sequence compared to other unrelated A/J Ig molecules (Capra *et al.*, 1977). The primary structure of phosphocholine-binding (MOPC603, TEPC15, MOPC167), inulin-binding (EPC109, Aml, ABPC-4, UPC61 and 47N), and galactan-binding (J533, XRPC24, XRPC44, J601) myeloma proteins provided new insight into the relationship between Id determinants and complementary-determining hypervariable regions (Vrana *et al.*, 1978; Potter *et al.*, 1977, 1979; Claflin and Davie, 1975a; Rudikoff and Potter, 1974; Kabat *et al.*, 1979). Recently, Clevinger *et al.* (1980) determined the complete sequence of several monoclonal antibodies specific for $\alpha(1\rightarrow3)$dextran. They found that the structure of J5581dX is located in the second hypervariable region, whereas that of IdI is in the third hypervariable region. These findings taken collectively clearly show a close relationship between combining site, hypervariable region, and idiotypes. However, a second family of Id determinants clearly have as structural correlates the framework segments of the V region of Ig molecules.

V. V_H-V_L Idiotypic Determinants

An important aspect of localization of Id determinants was to establish the contribution of heavy and light chains to the expression of idiotypic specificity borne by native antibody molecules. These were already evident by both precipitin analyses in agar gel and by hemagglutination inhibition experiments. Anti-idiotypic antisera were more readily obtained against λ light chains than against H type. Few workers have succeeded in obtaining anti-idiotypic antisera by immunization with isolated heavy chains. In the studies with anti-Id antisera made against whole human myeloma proteins, the bulk of antisera required both combinations of H and L chains for idiotypic expression (Kunkel, 1970).

However, in few exceptional cases it was reported that certain Id determinants borne by native myeloma proteins could be expressed by either light or heavy chains alone (Grey et al., 1965; Wang et al., 1970).

Recently, this problem was studied using murine myeloma proteins. Lieberman et al. (1977) prepared hybrid molecules between H and L chains of six inulin-binding myeloma proteins with H or L chains of XRPC24, which is a galactan-binding myeloma protein, to establish the topography of major IdXs. This study showed that a specific V$_H$V$_L$ pair is needed for the expression of IdX. Five out of these six inulin-binding myeloma proteins are determined by light chains, since they exert a dominant influence on the degree of affinity between the protein and fructosan trisaccharide. In contrast, heavy chains make major contributions in the case of ABPC4 inulin-binding myeloma proteins. These data are in agreement with those obtained by Streefkerk et al. (1978), in which the binding affinity of heterologous H-L chaing recombinants derived from monoclonal murine inulin binding myeloma proteins was studied. Eichmann (1978) has also studied the reactivity of four guinea pig anti-A5A Id sera versus the hybrid molecules reconstructed from H and L chains of A5A antibodies and from pooled mouse IgG. Two of these antisera reacted preferentially with A5A H chains and two others with A5A L chains. It should be mentioned that in this study the reconstructed hybrids between the H chain of A5A and the L chain of normal mouse Ig as well as L-A5A : H-normal Ig failed to exhibit binding activity for A-CHO Streptococcus A antigen as the native A5A molecule, despite the fact that they continued to react with these four, selected anti-Id antibodies. Both heavy and light chains are needed for the expression of IdX borne by MOPC173 (Schiff et al., 1973), J558 (Carson and Weigert, 1973), TEPC15 (Claflin and Rudihoff, 1979) myeloma proteins. Therefore, the majority of these findings suggest that specific associations between H and L chains are required for the expression of both antigen binding activity and idiotypic specificities. However, in certain situations the contribution of one or another chain to the idiotype specificity could be dominant. A similar conclusion was drawn from the genetic studies of idiotype expression in recombinant inbred strains of mice (Lieberman *et al.*, 1977; Jack *et al.*, 1977).

VI. Polymorphism of Idiotypes

It is well known that the majority of antigens induce a heterogeneous response, a manifestation of the stimulation of different clones by the same antigenic determinants. Since the idiotypes are phenotypic markers of V region genes, several investigators focused their efforts on the investigation of the distribution of IdX in the products of various clones. The conclusion of various observations and experimental findings is that idiotypic systems are polymorphic.

A. Expression of Idiotypes on Various Clones

Serological and isoelectric focusing (IEF) studies led Davie and his co-workers to estimate that a minimum of five clones are involved in the response to $\alpha(1\rightarrow3)$dextran (Hansburg *et al.*, 1976, 1977). Three of these clones bore IdI of J558, MOPC104, and U102 myeloma proteins, as well as J558IdX; one clone which expressed IdX lacked the three IdIs and one was deficient in IdX. The IEF analysis indicated very clearly that there are various clonotypes which express IdX of $\alpha(1\rightarrow3)$dextran-binding myeloma proteins in BALB/c, BAB14, and C58J mice.

Eichmann (1974) studied the expression of A5AIdX on anti-A-CHO polysaccharide antibodies in several individual A/J mice following immunization with *Streptococcus* A. A5AId$^+$ antibodies appeared to be represented by two to four bands which were stained with ^{131}I-labeled A-CHO. However, IEF patterns of the sera from various individual A/He mice indicated that not all spectrotypes representing A5AIdX had an identical pI. Therefore, it appeared that A5AId is shared by a family of closely related clones in A/J mice.

In other antigenic systems Mäkelä and his co-workers (Imanishi and Mäkelä, 1973; Mäkelä and Imanishi, 1975) studied a fine specificity related idiotype expressed on anti-NP antibodies of C57BL/6 mice, controlled by a V_H gene linked to *Ig-1^b* allotype. After immunization with NP, the mice produced heteroclitic anti-NP antibodies which had two to nine times higher affinity for NIP- and NNP-related haptens than for immunogenic hapten. The V-h^{NP} marker has been shown to be associated with the N1, N2, N3, and N4 isoelectric focusing pattern (McMichel *et al.,* 1975). This V-h^{NP} marker appears to be heterogeneous, since two to four genes seem to be involved (Mäkelä *et al.,* 1977). Indeed, anti-NPId antibodies cross-react with N2, N3, and N4 spectrotypes but with different affinity. Recently, we have shown (Bona *et al.,* 1979d) that the IgG anti-inulin antibodies elicited by immunization of BALB/c mice with bacterial levan and which are represented by four bands can be removed by precipitation with anti-IdX B or G antibodies (Fig. 1.1). A restricted heterogeneity spectrotype pattern was observed in the anti-allotype (IgG$_{2a}^{b}$) antibody response. The anti-allotype antibody response against the b allelic form of IgG$_2$, is under *Ir* gene control but independent of *Igh-C* genetic markers.

The anti-allotype antibodies produced by responder strains of *d, b, r, p, g* and *s* H-2 type expressed a IdX which seems to be under the control of a closely related family of *V* genes (Bona *et al.,* 1980b).

A very similar spectrotypic pattern was observed in all the strains of mice which produced IdX-bearing anti-allotype antibody, with the exception of RIII and 129/sv. mice. The study of the spectrotype of the IgG anti-phosphocholine antibody response in BALB/c mice showed a very striking similarity in all individuals of this strain. The anti-phosphocholine antibody response in BALB/c mice is characterized by a dominant T15Id which is expressed on more than 90% of the anti-phosphocholine antibodies (Cosenza and Kohler, 1972). The molecular uniformity of the T15$^+$ anti-phosphocholine response was determined by the study of the IEF patterns with four different anti-T15 sera (Claflin and Cubberley, 1978).

The above-mentioned findings indicate that the same idiotypic determinants can be shared by the products of various clones, and that the same *V* region genes can be expressed on the products of various clones with the same antigenic specificity.

B. Expression of Idiotype on Various Classes of Ig

The presence of the same idiotypic determinants on antibodies belonging to various Ig classes represents another aspect of heterogeneity of idiotypes. Oudin and Michel (1969a) showed that rabbit

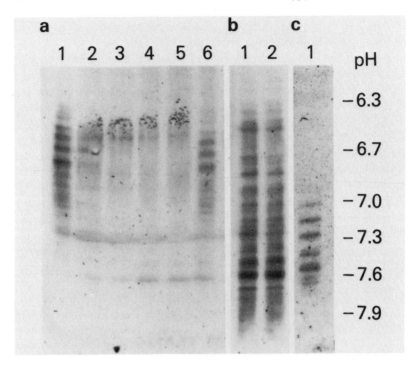

Fig. 1.1. Isoelectric focusing pattern of anti-inulin antiserum preincubated with anti-idiotype antibodies. (a) BALB/c anti-inulin pooled serum (25 μl) obtained from five individual mice 7 days after immunization with inulin-BA. Sera were preincubated for 1 hr with (1) 25 μl normal A/He serum, (2) μl A/He anti-T803 idiotype antiserum, (3) 50 μl A/He anti-T803 idiotype antiserum, (4) 25 μl A/He anti-E109 idiotype antiserum, (5) 50 μl A/He anti-E109 idiotype antiserum, (6) 25 μl A/He anti-MOPC384 idiotype antiserum. (b) C57BL/Ka anti-inulin serum (25 μl) obtained 7 days after immunization with inulin-KLH preincubated with (1) 25 μl normal A/He serum, (2) 25 μl A/He anti-E109 idiotype antiserum. (c) BALB/c anti-dextran (B512) serum treated with 25 μl A/He anti-E109 idiotype antiserum. The radioactive overlay consisted of [¹²⁵I]dextran and the film was exposed 2 days.

IgM and IgG anti-*S. typhi* antibodies shared the same Id determinants. In fact, an homologous anti-Id antibody cannot discriminate between IgM or IgG anti-*S. typhi* antibody. Oudin correctly interpreted these results in 1969, considering that the antibody molecules which carry the same idiotypic specificity in two Ig classes are supposedly synthesized by the same cells or at least belong to the same cell line. Penn *et al.* (1970) reported that in the case of a myeloma serum, the same antigenic individual specificities were shared between IgG and IgM. Fu *et al.* (1975) have shown that surface IgD and IgM of leukemic lymphocytes were stained by an anti-Id antibody obtained by immunization with a monoclonal IgM K band isolated from the serum of this leukemia patient.

After Oudin's observation in the case of anti-*S. typhi* antibody and Penn and Kunkel in the case of myeloma proteins, numerous reports have shown that the same idiotypic determinants are shared by various Ig classes, clearly indicating that the product of the same variable gene can be associated with the products of various constant genes (Wang *et al.*, 1970).

In further studies it was shown that J558IdX as well as M104E IdI of $\alpha(1\rightarrow3)$dextran-binding myeloma protein are expressed on 7 and 19 S anti-dextran antibodies in various strains of mice (Hansburg *et al.*, 1977). Claflin and Cubberley (1978) demonstrated that IgG_1, IgG_2, and IgG_3 anti-phosphocholine antibodies, which were induced following immunization with phosphocholine-KLH, expressed T15IdX. Ju *et al.* (1979b) likewise reported that cGAT IdX was expressed on IgM, IgG_1, and IgG_2 anti-GAT antibodies. Imanishi *et al.*, (1975) have found that NP idiotype was expressed in three Ig classes.

Similarly, the same *V* gene markers can be expressed not only on various classes of humoral antibodies but also on various classes of surface and intracytoplasma Ig, as was shown in the studies on myeloma patients (Fu *et al.*, 1975; Salsano *et al.*, 1974; Schroer *et al.*, 1974).

C. Common Idiotype on Antibodies with Distinct Specificities

Since the discovery of idiotypic determinants on myeloma proteins by Slater *et al.* (1955), it was accepted as a general rule that an idiotype is associated only with antibody molecules of a given specificity but not with antibodies possessing different binding activity.

An intriguing aspect of the polymorphism of idiotypes was the discovery of idiotypic determinants on antibodies with specificities for closed antigens or with unknown antibody function. Oudin and Cazenave (1971) have studied the expression of Id determinants of rabbit anti-hen ovalbumin antibodies. They found that idiotypic specificity was common to three families of antibodies.

1. Anti-hen ovalbumin antibodies eluted from immunoadsorbants by different concentrations of $MgCl_2$. In these eluted fractions, two or three idiotypes were detected by immunodiffusion analysis

2. Antibodies which reacted only with hen, hen and turkey, or hen, turkey, and duck ovalbumin

3. Antibodies devoid of anti-ovalbumin activity

Eichmann *et al.* (1977), in a study of the frequency of A5AId[+] anti-*Streptococcus* A antibody-forming cells, observed a tenfold increase in the number of A5AId-bearing B cells after priming with A-CHO-streptococcal polysaccharide. Surprisingly, only about one-half of these B lymphocytes have been specific for A-CHO. Recently, we have shown that we can identify in the sera of young BALB/c mice molecules which share the IdXA of inulin-binding myeloma proteins but which lack detectable inulin-binding activity (Bona *et al.*, 1978).

In BALB/c mice IdX-G-A and B bearing anti-inulin antibodies occur late, at day 28 after birth (Bona *et al.*, 1978). However, we observed in the sera of 1- or 2-week-old BALB/c mice molecules which bore IdXA. The concentration of these IdXA-bearing molecules was not increased following immunization with bacterial levan or inulin-BA and was not altered by adsorption on inulin immunoadsorbants. These results indicated that the IdXA[+]-bearing molecules of young BALB/c mice have not been produced by anti-inulin antibody forming cells. It is possible that these molecules are synthesized by a protoclone expressed in young animals from which derive in adult animals, the clones secreting IdXA,-B, and -G bearing anti-inulin antibodies.

Another aspect of the polymorphism of idiotype expression is the presence of idiotypic determinants on antibody molecules with different antigenic specificities. Cazenave and Oudin (1973) observed that antibodies against human fibrinogen shared the idiotypic determinants of antibodies obtained following immunization with two fragments of native fibrinogen obtained by splitting with plasmin.

Karol *et al.* (1978) have also shown that idiotypic determinants of goat anti-sickle cell hemoglobin (i.e., anti-Val antibodies) were shared by an antibody population that bind to human adult hemoglobin (HbA[cr]).

Recently, we have shown that anti-Id antibodies against a BALB/c anti-IgG$_{2a}^{b}$ allotype antibodies reacted with monoclonal antibodies specific for CH2 and CH3 domains of the Fc fragment of IgG$_{2a}^{b}$ (Bona *et al.*, 1980b).

Of six monoclonal antibodies studied, two were specific for CH3 and one for CH2 domains of the Fc fragment of the b allelic form of IgG_{2a} (Tables 1.7 and 1.8).

Recently, Ju *et al.* (1980) detected shared GTGL idiotype on antibodies with distinct antigenic specificity in various mouse strains. Indeed, these authors found that antibodies specific for GAT or GLφ copolymers and antibodies with a dual specificity for GAT and GLφ expressed GTGL idiotype.

Several explanations can be entertained concerning the sharing of Id determinants by antibodies recognizing different antigenic specificities.

1. Antibodies which share IdX, although they have a different specificity, are directed toward the same antigenic site. Karol *et al.* (1978) considered this explanation plausible for the shared idiotypes between goat anti-Val and anti-HbA^{cr} antibodies. Indeed, anti-Val and anti-HbA^{cr} share a number of amino acid residues complementary to a number of amino acids on sickle cell hemoglobin among which a key residue is the B^6-position. Most of amino acid side chains of anti-Val and anti-HbA^{cr} molecules are identical, whereas one side chain is different. According to these authors, the side chain difference is responsible for the differences in the observed binding specificity of anti-Val and anti-HbA^{cr} antibodies, whereas the shared residues can be responsible for the strong idiotype cross reactivity.

2. Another hypothesis which can explain the presence of idiotypic determinants on antibodies with distinct specificities is that these antibodies are encoded by two separate germ line genes which derive from one ancestral gene by duplication and then undergone independent evolutionary pressure. Alternatively, a *V* region gene can arise by a somatic mutation from other genes or the germ line gene of the common ancestor and the antigens selectively stimulate the mutant clone.

3. It is also possible that by a recombination of *V-J* the same *V* gene product can be expressed on antibodies with distinct antigen binding specificities. This hypothesis can be supported by the interesting results reported by Schilling *et al.* (1980), which showed that monoclonal anti α(1→3)dextran antibodies and some myeloma proteins bearing different specificities possess identical J segments.

4. Finally, the presence of common idiotypes on antibody molecules with distinct antigen-binding specificity might be explained by insertion of mini genes. Indeed, it appears possible that DNA segments

TABLE 1.7

Properties of Hybridoma Anti-IgG$_{2a}^b$ Allotype Antibody[a]

Hybridoma	Immunized donors	Specificity of hybridoma product	Specificity for Fc domains	Ig class of hybridoma product	HA titer (ln)	
					CBPC101[c]	C57BL/6 Ig[r]
10–3.6	CW.B	IA.17	—	G$_{2a}$	0	0
Ig(1b)5.7.1	BALB/c	IgG$_{2a}^b$	CH3	G$_3$	12	>12
Ig(1b)3.1	BALB/c	IgG$_{2a}^b$	CH3	G$_1$	11	10
Ig(1b)2.9	BALB/c	IgG$_{2a}^b$	CH2	G$_{2a}$	12	>12
Ig(1b)4.7	SJA	IgG$_{2a}^b$	Hinge	G$_1$	0	0
S1G.1E	BALB/c	IgG$_{2a}^b$	ND[b]	G$_1$	24	24
S1A.1A	BALB/c	IgG$_{2a}^b$	ND	G$_1$	24	24
BALB/c anti-CBPC101 antibody	BALB/c	IgG$_{2a}^b$	ND	ND	12	16

[a] From Bona et al., 1980b.
[b] Not done.
[c] SRBC.

TABLE 1.8

Study of IdX Expression on Hybridoma Anti-IgG$_{2a}^b$ Allotype Antibodies Using BAB.14 Anti-Id[a]

	HI titer (ln); SRBC coated with anti-CBPC101 antibody from				Inhibition of RIA[b] using ^{3}H-labeled anti-CBPC101 antibody from			
Hybridoma No.	BALB/c	C.AL20	P/J	DBA/2	BALB/c	C.AL20	P/J	DBA/2
Ig(1b)5.7.1	>8	>8	5	4	100[c]	1000	10	10
Ig(1b)3.1	5	ND[d]	ND	ND	100	ND	ND	ND
Ig(1b)2.9	4	2	2	>8	>300	10	10	30
Ig(1b)4.7	0	ND	ND	ND	<3	ND	ND	ND
S1G.1E	2	>8	2	>8	3	100	<10	30
S1A.1A	2	>8	4	>8	10	30	<10	100
10–3.6	0	0	0	0	<3	ND	ND	ND

[a] From Bona et al., 1980b.

[b] RIA, radioimmunoassay.

[c] Results are reported as the reciprocal of the greatest dilution of hybridoma product which gave greater than 50% inhibition of binding of ^{3}H-labeled anti-allotype antibody to plates coated with a 1 : 50,000 dilution of BAB.14 anti-(BALB/c anti-CBPC101) antiserum. Dilutions tested were 1 : 3, 1 : 10, 1 : 30, 1 : 100, 1 : 300, 1 : 1000, and 1 : 3000.

[d] Not done.

encoding the cross-reactive idiotypic determinants (mini gene) could be incorporated into two separate V genes responsible for the synthesis of two antibodies with different specificities.

Therefore, numerous data clearly indicate great polymorphism in the idiotypic system. The V region genes which encode the idiotypic specificity can be expressed on various clones which produce antibodies with the same specificity but different affinity and which belongs to various Ig classes. In addition, a common Id can be identified on antibodies with various antigenic specificity or unknown antibody activity. Of course, the expression of the same V region genes in various clones represents strong evidence of germ line gene origins of IdXs. By contrast, IdI, which is associated with a unique V sequence and which is not inherited, could be the result of a somatic mutational process.

The polymorphism of IdX indicates that the concept of one structural gene–one idiotype as a V region marker is not valid. Indeed, several germ line genes or a closely related family of V region genes could be responsible for the heterogeneity of IdXs.

VII. Genetics of Idiotypes

During the last year, several excellent reviews had as their subject the genetic control of expression of idiotypes (Eichmann, 1975b; Mäkelä et al., 1977; Weigert and Riblet, 1978, Potter, 1977). However, for practical purposes related to the presentation of the cellular basis of idiotypy, we would like to mention briefly the genetics of various IdXs studied in mice.

Genetic analysis of the expression of IdXs in mice and other species has revealed that they are inherited according to Mendelian rules. Some, but not all, expressions of IdXs are controlled by C-h genes which determine the specificity of allotypes. Mendelian inheritance of idiotypes was determined in breeding experiments, and the linkage to allotypes was established by studying the distribution of idiotypes and allotypes among the F_1, F_2, and backcross progeny as well as various recombinant inbred mice. Recombinant mice were obtained by breeding experiments in which a few genetically stable markers in a newly generated linkage were selected. The recombination was considered established when the new genetic marker combination was stable and inherited in a Mendelian fashion.

However, in some antibody responses the expression of IdX appears to be under the control of Ir genes, since the ability to make antibodies in certain strains of mice is Ir gene determined. This is the case of the anti-nuclease antibody response (Lozner et al., 1974) and of the ability to synthesize anti-allotype antibodies. Only mice bearing a, b, p, r, and s haplotypes are able to produce antibody specific for the a allele for IgA (Lieberman and Humphrey, 1971), and those with b, p, r, s and v H-2 types produce antibody specific for the a allele of IgG_{2a} (Lieberman and Humphrey, 1972).

An IdX was detected only on anti-IgG_{2a}^b allotype antibody of d, b, p, r, g, and s H-2 types since only these haplotypes are able to produce anti-allotype antibodies (Bona et al., 1980b) (Table 1.6).

The more extensively studied V region phenotypic markers are listed as shown below.

$T15IdX$. Expressed on several IgA_k-phosphocholine-binding myeloma proteins of BALB/c mice as TEPC15, HOPC8, S107, S63, and MOPC299, as well as on anti-phosphocholine antibodies produced following immunization with R36A pneumococcal vaccine and T-dependent phosphocholine conjugates. The expression of T15IdX is linked to Ig-1^a allotype at the humoral level (Lieberman et al.) but at the cellular level can be detected in mice bearing $Ig-1^b$ allotype (Cancro *et al.*, 1977).

IdXG,B, and A of anti-inulin antibodies. Expressed on $\beta(2\rightarrow1)$ and $\beta(2\rightarrow6)$fructosan-binding myeloma proteins and anti-inulin antibodies produced in response to immunization with bacterial levan and inulin conjugates (Bona *et al.*, 1978). The expression of these idiotypes is linked to $Ig-1^a$. However, in other studies of mice, such as DBA/2 (Ig-1^c), A/He and AL/N (Ig-1^a), and CAL20 (Ig-1^a), these IdXs were expressed (Lieberman *et al.*, 1977) (Table 1.9).

J558IdX. Expressed on J558 and MOPC104E myeloma proteins and on antibodies of BALB/c mice elicited by immunization with $\alpha(1\rightarrow3)$dextran. Its expression is linked to $Ig-1^a$ allotype (Carson and Weigert, 1973).

IdX of galactan myeloma proteins. XRPC24, XRPC40, and T601, for example, originating from BALB/c mice is shared by anti-$\beta(1\rightarrow6)$D-galactan antibodies produced by mice bearing either $Ig-1^a$ or $Ig-1^b$ allotypes (Potter *et al.*, 1979).

460IdX. Shared by MOPC460-DNP binding myeloma proteins and anti-DNP or -TNP antibodies produced by mice bearing $Ig-1^a$ allotype (Zeldis *et al.*, 1979; Cazenave *et al.*, 1980).

S117IdX. Shared by S117 (IgA$_k$) myeloma proteins specific for

TABLE 1.9

Expression of IdXG, B, and A of Inulin-Binding Myeloma Proteins in Various Strains of Mice

Strain of mice	Igh-V	Igh-C	H-2	IdX		
				G	B	A
BALB/c	a	a	d	+	+	+
RICXBG	a	a	b	+	+	+
RICXBJ	a	a	b	+	+	+
BC.8	a	a	b	+	+	+
BAB14	a	b	d	+	+	−
A/He	e	e	a	+	+	+
CAL.20	d	d	d	+	+	+
C58J	a	a	k	+	+	+
RIII	g	g	r	+	−	+
AKR	d	d	k	−	−	−
CBA	J	J	k	−	−	−
DBA/2	c	c	d	−	−	−

A-CHO polysaccharide antigen of *Streptococcus* A and anti-*Streptococcus* A antibodies produced by Ig-1^a mice. *N*-Acetylglucosamine is the dominant sugar of A-CHO antigens (Berek *et al.*, 1976).

A5AIdX. The idiotype of clone A5A which secretes antibodies specific for *N*-acetylglucosamine, the dominant sugar of A-CHO antigen, and which was obtained in 1972 by Eichmann by *in vivo* spleen cloning in A/J mice. The A5A IdX is expressed on anti-*Streptococcus* A antibodies elicited from A/J mice which bear *Ig-1^e* allotype. The genes coding for S117 IdX are linked to *Ig-1^a* and those coding for A5AIdX are linked to *Ig-1^e*. These appear to be alleles which control the synthesis of antibodies specific for A-CHO. However, the expression of A5A and S117 IdX in mice bearing *Ig-1^e* allotype suggests a pseudoallelic relationship between different haplotypes which permits the expression of the same gene in an allelic or nonallelic manner (Berek *et al.*, 1976).

Ars IdX. Shared by anti-arsonate antibodies elicited in the mice bearing *Ig-1^e* allotype following immunization with *p*-azophenylarsonate (Nisonoff *et al.*, 1977). Other haptens from the arsonate family induce an inherited IdX as *p*-azobenzenearsonate (ABA) and ABA coupled to *p*-hydroxyphenylacetic acid (ABA-HOP) Mäkelä *et al.*, 1977). ABA IdX is linked to *Ig-1^e* haplotype, whereas ABA-HOPIdX was identified in mice strains bearing either *Ig-1^e* or *Ig-1^b* haplotypes.

Nuclease IdX. Found on antibodies produced by BALB/c mice after immunization with staphylococcal nuclease. This idiotype was found in anti-nuclease antibodies produced by A/J (Ig-1^e) and SJL (Ig-1^b) mice (Fathman *et al.*, 1977).

V_{HNP^b}Id. Mice of strains C57BL/6, LP, or 101 immunized with carrier conjugated with NP haptens produce anti-NP antibody. The affinity of these anti-NP antibodies is higher for NNP or NIP related haptens than for NP immunizing haptens. These kinds of antibodies were called "heteroclitic" antibodies. Anti-NP^b idiotype antibodies also react with heteroclitic antibodies. The expression of the V_{HNP^b} phenotypic marker is controlled by *Ig-1^b* genes (Mäkelä *et al.*, 1977).

TMA-Id. The expression of IdX of anti-TMA antibodies is controlled by *Ig-1^e* genes (Alevy *et al.*, 1980).

CGATIdX. Anti-GAT antibodies of all mouse strains, including both responder and nonresponder strains, express a common idiotype(s) called cGAT (Ju *et al.*, 1978a). The "GT" antigenic moiety of the GAT molecule is responsible for the induction of GAT antibodies which express the cGATIdX (Ju *et al.,* 1979a). By contrast, antibodies specific for "GA" antigenic molecules produced during the response following immunization with GAT represent a minor family of antibodies which bear an unrelated IdX called GA-1, which is an interstrain IdX (Ju *et al.,* 1979a).

The genes which control the expression of IdX's are structural *V* region germ line genes. Their Mendelian manner of inheritance and their distribution among all individuals and on various Ig classes support their germ line origin. However, the mechanism of their expression and activation is still unclear.

The polymorphism of the idiotypic system clearly indicates that idiotypic determinants expressed on various clonotypes could be the products of several structural genes. Whether this closely related family of *V* genes, which encodes the IdXs, is inherited as a cluster remains to be established by a more direct approach.

VIII. Control of Expression of the Silent Idiotypic Repertoire

The understanding of mechanism(s) which control the expression of IdX represents one of the most important aspects of genetics of idiotypy. Several recent findings indicate that a significant fraction of the immune repertoire is silent in the mammalian species. However, this silent repertoire can be activated by adequate immunological manipulation. Thus, DBA/2 mice are unable to make $460Id^+$ anti-TNP antibodies, since the expression of 460Id is controlled by $Ig-1^a$ genes. However, these mice immunized with anti-460Id antibodies in order to produce anti-(anti-460Id) antibodies and then with TNP-Ficoll made anti-TNP antibodies bearing 460Id (Cazenave *et al.,* 1980) (Fig. 1.2).

Similarly, in genetically unrelated rabbits a silent clone expressing the Id of anti-RNase or anti-*Micrococcus* polysaccharide antibodies has been activated following intentional immunization to produce anti-(anti-Id) antibodies (Cazenave, 1977; Urbain *et al.,* 1977).

The stimulation of silent clones can be obtained not only by induction of anti-(anti-Id) antibodies but also by idiotype suppression. In several antigenic systems it has been shown that the suppression of major or dominant IdXs leads to the expression of silent or minor clones. Thus, Augustin and Cosenza (1976) have shown that after

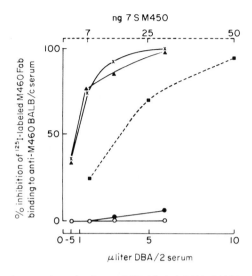

Fig. 1.2. Inhibition of the binding of ^{125}I-labeled I-Fab M460 to BALB/c anti-M460 idiotype antibodies: 7 S M460 protein (■--■--■); sera from two normal DBA/2 mice immunized against DNP-ovalbumin (O———O, ●———●): sera from two DBA/2 mice preimmunized against homogeneous anti-M460 antibody F6(51) and subsequently immunized against DNP-ovalbumin (▲———▲, X − X): this inhibition is no longer observed if anti-DNP antibodies are removed on DNP-lysine-Sepharose. From Cazenave *et al.,* 1980.

neonatal suppression of the T15IdX$^+$ antibody response, which represents more than 90% of the total, anti-phosphocholine response is replaced by a T15IdX$^-$ anti-phosphocholine response.

In nude BALB/c mice the suppression of IdXs borne by anti-inulin antibodies was followed by the occurrence of anti-levan antibodies bearing 48Id when these mice have been immunized with bacterial levan. In normal BALB/c mice the A48Id cannot be detected in anti-levan antibodies (Lieberman *et al.,* 1979). Recently, it was shown that neonatal treatment with 10 ng anti-A48Id antibodies led to highly significant increase of A48Id$^+$ component of anti-bacterial levan response (Hiernaux *et al.,* 1981).

In the rabbit, Brown *et al.* (1979) have also shown that the occurrence of anti-Id auto antibodies during immunization with *Micrococcus lysodeikticus* polysaccharide coincided with the appearance of new clonotypes. These had not been observed in preimmune serum or in the serum obtained after first immunization.

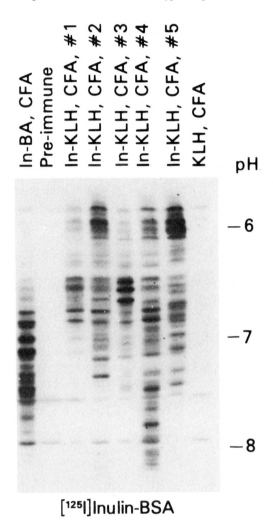

Fig. 1.3. Isoelectric focusing pattern of BALB/c anti-inulin (In) antibodies raised against In conjugates. The anti-In-BA serum is a pool prepared from the sera obtained from three BALB/c mice at 10 days after immunization with In-BA. The preimmune and anti-KLH sera were from pools prepared from sera obtained from 10 BALB/c mice before immunization or 10 days after immunization with KLH. Anti-In-KLH sera were obtained from five individual BALB/c mice 1 week after the third immunization with In-KLH. Sera were focused, and the gel was exposed to [^{125}I]inulin-BSA.

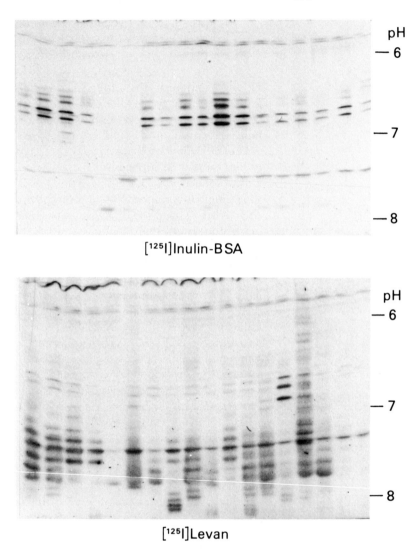

$[^{125}I]$Inulin-BSA

$[^{125}I]$Levan

Fig. 1.4. Isoelectric focusing pattern of BALB/c anti-BL antibodies. Sera obtained from 18 individual BALB/c mice at 10 days after immunization with BL were focused in duplicate gels in the same sample slot in both gels. The upper panel shows the antibodies reactive with $[^{125}I]$inulin-BSA, and the lower panel shows the antibodies reactive with ^{125}I-labeled BL.

Finally, new clonotypes can be activated by varying the presentation of antigens. Thus, Stein *et al.* (1980) showed that in BALB/c mice the IgG anti-inulin antibody response elicited by immunization with bacterial levan showed a very restricted IEF pattern. Only three to five bands bind [125I]-labeled bovine serum albumin(BSA)-inulin. The same number of bands have been observed after immunization with inulin NWSM conjugate and a highly heterogenous IEF pattern was observed after immunization with inulin-*B. abortus* or inulin-keyhole limpet heteroglutinin(KLH)conjugates (Fig. 1.3).

These findings indicate that the real idiotypic repertoire is much greater and this is revealed by the appearance of new clonotypes in

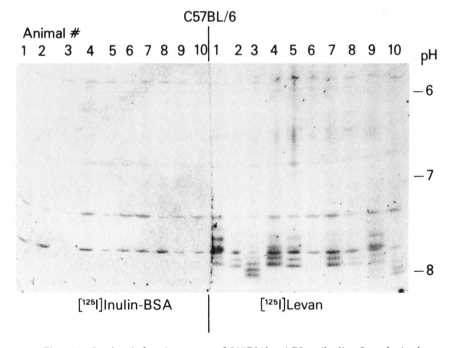

Fig. 1.5.   Isoelectric focusing pattern of C57BL/6 anti-BL antibodies. Sera obtained from 10 individual C57BL/6 mice at 10 days after immunization with BL were focused in duplicate in the same gel. The gel was cut and one-half was exposed to [125I]-inulin-BSA (left panel) and the other half to [125I]-BL (right panel). The bands seen on the left half of the gel (In overlay) are bands that we consider to represent nonspecific binding because the identical pattern can be seen with sera from unimmunized mice, as well as with immune sera, and with virtually any iodinated antigen that we have examined. No effort has been made to eliminate these bands as they serve as a useful internal marker.

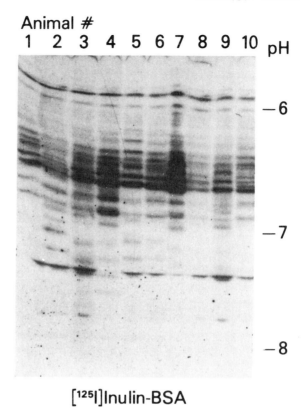

Animal #

Fig. 1.6. Isoelectric focusing pattern of (BALB/c × C57BL/6) F₁ anti-BL antibodies. Sera obtained from 10 individual (BALB/c × C57BL/6)F₁ mice at 10 days after immunization with BL were focused and exposed to [¹²⁵I]inulin-BSA.

animals previously suppressed or manipulated to produce anti-(anti-Id) antibodies or which have been immunized with hapten conjugates.

The existence of a silent repertoire suggests that the expression of some structural *V* genes which encode the IdX specificities can be under the control of regulatory genes. We have encountered an example of such regulatory genes in studying the genetic regulation of IEF patterns of the IgG anti-inulin response. The structural genes which control this response map to the *Ig-V* region of the *Igh* gene. The complexity of the IEF pattern of the IgG anti-inulin response requires genes found in the *a* (BALB/c) type of the *Igh* complex, but the expression of silent clones is regulated by at least one *C57BL*

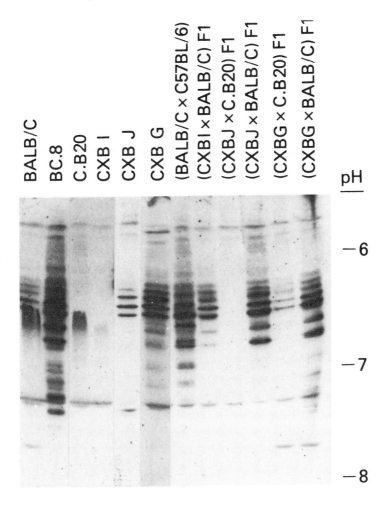

Fig. 1.7.　Isoelectric focusing pattern of anti-BL antibodies of different strains of mice. Sera obtained from representative individual mice (at least 10 individuals of each strain and 4 of each F_1 combination were examined) of various strains at 5 or 10 days after immunization with BL were focused and overlaid with [^{125}I]inulin-BSA.

gene. This regulatory gene designated by Stein *et al.* (1980) as spectrotype regulatory gene (*SR-1*) is not linked to the *Igh* gene complex, the major histocompatibility complex (MHC), or to genes controlling coat color.

In contrast to BALB/c mice, which after immunization with BL produce a high titer of IdX$^+$ anti-inulin antibodies and restricted IgG anti-inulin antibodies, the C57BL/6 mice show a weak titer of IdX$^-$ anti-inulin antibody and no IgG anti-inulin (Figs. 1.4 and 1.5). However, the (BALB/c × C57BL/6)F$_1$ hybrids all developed a vigorous IdX$^+$ anti-inulin response, and IEF analysis revealed a more heterogeneous pattern than anti-inulin antibodies produced in BALB/c mice immunized with BL or with inulin coupled with various carriers (Fig. 1.6). It seems that the increased heterogeneity of the IgG anti-inulin response is not related to the expression of a latent anti-inulin response of the Igh^b type since the BC8 and CXBG RI anti-inulin antibodies express a degree of antibody heterogeneity greater than that of the F$_1$ anti-inulin antibodies (Fig. 1.7). Both BC8 and CXBG are Igh^a mice and H-2^b type. Analysis of the distribution of the heterogeneous IEF pattern in backcross (BALB/c × C57BL 6) × BALB/c progeny indicated that the C57BL/6 gene involved in regulation of the Igh^a anti-inulin response appears not to be linked to the *Igh* complex, to the MHC, or to the genes specifying coat color (Table 1.10). These data indicate that the expression of *Igh-V* structural

TABLE 1.10

Analysis of Backcross Mice[a]

		Spectrotype	
Trait		BALB/c-like	Non-BALB/c-like
Allotype	a/a	5	7
	a/b	5	7
H-2 type	d/d	7	6
	b/d	2	5
Sex	Male	4	6
	Female	6	9
Coat color	Albino	3	9
	Agouti	3	2
	Brown	4	4

[a] From Stein *et al.,* 1980.

genes of anti-inulin antibodies is under the control of non-allotype-linked background genes, such as *Sr-1,* which are present even in strains that lack the appropriate *Igh-V* genes themselves. Other studies on the recombinants of 129/SV × C57BL/6 and AL/N CAL.20 strains strongly suggest that such regulatory genes are not found exclusively in C57BL/6 mice.

These findings taken together suggest that an important fraction of the immune repertoire is silent. The activation of silent clones depends on various factors such as the presentation of antigens, the alteration of clonal dominance, the stimulation of anti-idiotypic responses, the suppressor cells and the regulatory genes which control the expression of Ig structural genes.

Ontogeny of Expression of Idiotypes

I. Scheme of Development of B Cells

The B cells and lymphomyeloid cells develop from pluripotential stem cells. The first stage of the differentiation process from stem cells is represented by large pre-B cells that later evolve into small pre-B cells. These small pre-B cells differentiate into immature B lymphocytes that finally give the virgin B lymphocytes. The virgin B lymphocytes stimulated by antigen or polyclonal B cell mitogens can differentiate into plasmoblast and plasma cells which are immunoglobulin (Ig)-secreting cells. The generation of the immune repertoire is dependent on the differentiation of these diverse populations of B lymphocytes which occur during ontogeny and which takes place at sites of hematopoiesis, especially in fetal liver.

There is little doubt that the B lymphocytes derive from pluripotential stem cells that are the ancestors of all blood cell types. Early histological studies have located the first B cells in regenerating spleens around periarteriolar sheets of white pulp area (Rozing *et al.,* 1977). It was therefore suggested that particular regions of bone marrow and spleen determine differentiation of cells, but the factors which drive this process are unknown. Therefore, pre-B cells probably derive from pluripotential stem cells. The first pre-B cells in irradiated reconstituted mice were found in bone marrow, but not seen in spleen colonies (CFU), in which myelopoiesis was the major activity (Owen, 1979).

The pre-B cells are rapidly dividing large lymphocytes which contain intracytoplasmic Ig but which lack surface Ig (sIg) as well as other surface receptors, such as Fc, C3, and mitogens (Cooper and Lawton,1979). These pre-B cells have been found in fetal liver and umbilical blood at 11 days of gestation (Raff *et al.,* 1976) but not in yolk sac cell preparation from 8 day gestation embryo. There remains some controversy concerning the presence of sIg on pre-B cells. Surface Ig was not detected with fluoresceinated or iodinated anti-IgM antibody. In view of the relative insensitivity of these techniques, however, up to 10,000 sIg molecules could exist on the pre-B cells. This might be the reason that the pre-B cells can rosette sheep red blood cells (SRBC) coated with anti-Ig antibodies (Rosenberg and Parish, 1977). However, in functional studies it was shown that the pre-B cells are not sensitive to the anti-Ig antibodies which did not induce the suppression of IgM synthesis or their differentiation into lymphocytes in a culture of fetal liver cells. If the pre-B cells have sIg, either they have a rapid turnover or their low density prevents the suppression induced by anti-IgM antibodies. The greatest number of pre-B cells are generated in the fetal liver.

Nondividing small lymphocytes derived from pre-B cells possess sIg and bear Fc receptors and Ia and $H-2^k$ antigens. The mature small lymphocytes bear sIgM and sIgD, Ia, and $H-2^k$ antigens and the receptors for Fc and C3 (Osmond, 1979). The first $sIgM^+$ B lymphocytes can be stimulated either by antigen or B cell mitogens to differentiate into plasma cells and to secrete Ig. Melchers *et al.* (1977) have detected IgM synthesis in fetal liver as early as day 11 of gestation, indicating that the differentiation of pre-B cells to virgin small lymphocytes is very early. The $sIgM^+$ small lymphocyte is particularly sensitive to anti-IgM-induced suppression and to tolerance induced by antigens. The factors responsible for differentiation of the pre-B cells in the immature and mature small lymphocytes are not known. However, the fact that only 25% of B lymphocytes were found in germ-free mice suggests that the environmental antigens could play an important role in the regulation of B lymphocyte differentiation (Osmond, 1979). Studies in humans support the notion that pre-B cells differentiate in hematopoietic foci of fetal liver and then migrate to the lymphoid organs (Gathings *et al.,* 1977).

In the rabbit it was reported that the lymphoblasts appear in the spleen after 20 days of gestation and small lymphocytes at 27–28 days (Archer *et al.*, 1964). At the time of birth the lymphocytes increase in number and spread into the splenic cords, and 4 days after birth they can be found in the appendix and the peripheral lymph nodes.

The pre-B cells were evident in rabbits and showed allelic exclusion of antibody synthesis. Interestingly, in allotype-suppressed F_1 hybrids the pre-B cells contained cytoplasmic Ig (cIg) bearing suppressed allotype, indicating that they were not sensitive to the suppressor function of maternal anti-allotype antibodies (Hayward *et al.*, 1978).

We have also found that the fetal liver cells of 17–29 day embryos do not express certain receptors since they cannot be stimulated to incorporate [^{3}H]thymidine by NWSM or anti-allotype antibodies (Table 2.1). Only when the pre-B cells migrate from the fetal liver into the spleen was the NWSM responsiveness acquired at 29 days of gestation. In 1-day-old newborn rabbits, the spleen lymphocytes exhibited the ability to respond to both NWSM and anti-allotype antibody.

The ability to synthesize Ig was first detected in 22-day fetal liver, but this synthesis cannot be increased by NWSM-polyclonal activator even in 23-day-old fetal liver cells. By contrast the Ig synthesis of 23-day embryonic and 1-day-old newborn spleen cells was significantly increased by NWSM (Table 2.2) (Cazenave *et al.*, 1978). These data suggest that pre-B cells are present very early in rabbit fetal liver, but they acquire the NWSM receptor only when they migrate into the spleen at 23 days of gestation. Only after birth do they express both the mitogen receptor and sIg so that they can be stimulated by NWSM as well as by anti-allotype antibodies.

Finally, in birds the pre-B cells are observed in bursa of Fabricius very early in ontogeny, and their differentiation into virgin lymphocyte takes place at this site (Cooper *et al.*, 1979).

II. Expression of Idiotypic Determinants in Pre-B Cells

There are very little data on the expression of the phenotypic markers of V-region genes in the pluripotential stem cells and in the early stages of ontogenic development of B cells.

Forni *et al.* (1979) have recently studied the expression of V region genes on the surface Ig$^-$ precursor of B cells in murine fetal liver and bone marrow. They reported that 0.7–1.2% of fetal liver and 3.6–

TABLE 2.1

Age Dependence Responsiveness to NWSM[a]

Origin of cells	Age of donor of cells	10⁶ Cells/ml incubated with NWSM			
		Nil (control)	1 μg	10 μg	100 μg
Fetal liver	17 days	1,622 ± 181[b]	1,053 ± 105	1,416 ± 153	1,102 ± 79
Fetal liver	22 days	3,546 ± 308	1,638 ± 287	961 ± 128	1,122 ± 144
Fetal spleen	22 days	695 ± 13	ND[c]	323 ± 18	ND
Fetal liver	26 days	9,024 ± 564	6,134 ± 587	4,661 ± 428	5,358 ± 545
Fetal liver	29 days	10,690 ± 677	4,432 ± 591	2,809 ± 398	3,898 ± 383
Fetal spleen	29 days	1,226 ± 385	ND	453 ± 15	ND
New born liver	1 day	4,385 ± 223	4,923 ± 61	4,473 ± 785	4,476 ± 780
New born spleen	1 day	1,651 ± 33	ND	15,628 ± 435	27,249 ± 1,018
Adult spleen	12 months	1,670 ± 226	5,870 ± 399	40,897 ± 1,395	65,015 ± 2,306

[a] From Cazenave et al., 1978

[b] cpm: mean of triplicate cultures ± S.D.

[c] Not done.

TABLE 2.2

Age Dependence of Synthesis of Immunoglobulin (b4 Allotype)[a]

Origin of cells	Age of donor of cells	Culture incubated with			
		Nil (control)	NWSM (100 μg)	Con A (50 μg)	PHA (10 μg)
Fetal liver	17 days	<100[b]	<100	<100	<100
Fetal liver	22 days	530 ± 30	310 ± 50	320 ± 30	400 ± 50
Fetal liver	26 days	530 ± 50	500 ± 50	450 ± 60	600 ± 90
Fetal liver	29 days	4,500 ± 250	3,800 ± 200	3,400 ± 180	3,600 ± 200
Fetal spleen	29 days	2,300 ± 150	12,300 ± 2,200	ND[c]	ND
Newborn liver	1 day	<100	<100	<100	<100
Newborn spleen	1 day	780 ± 50	14,250 ± 750	975 ± 75	605 ± 125
Adult spleen	12 months	15,600 ± 4,440	42,000 ± 6,000	3,900 ± 100	5,400 ± 200

[a] From Cazenave et al., 1978.
[b] Nanograms per culture. Each culture contained 25 × 10^6 cells and 5 ml medium.
[c] Not done.

4.1% of bone marrow cells were stained with four anti-Id antibodies specific for J558, MOPC460, W3123, and TEPC15 idiotypes. These anti-Id antibodies recognize and interact with V-region-like structures expressed on a non-Ig receptor of precursors of pre-B cells. Accordingly, anti-Id antibodies would have an important role in the regulation and differentiation of precursor B cells by their binding to mitogen and/or growth receptors. Coutinho *et al.* (1978) have shown that the pretreatment of Ig⁻ cells with anti-J558Id antibodies and complement (C) prevented the ability of lipopolysaccharide (LPS) to stimulate the polyclonal differentiation of Ig⁻ cells into Ig-secreting cells. By contrast, preincubation of Ig⁻ cells with anti-J558Id antibodies without C for a few days led to a marked enhancement of LPS-induced Ig-secreting cells. Coutinho *et al.* (1978) considered that the mitogen receptor can share Id determinants with humoral antibodies and therefore the anti-Id antibodies can exhibit mitogen-like properties.

A number of criticisms can be raised against these results. The staining technique used in these experiments consisted of TNP-labeled anti-Id antibodies revealed by fluoresceinated rabbit anti-TNP antibodies. Since this staining can be due to the binding of one or two antibodies by Fc receptors of Ig⁻ cells, the utilization of $F(ab')_2$ fragments of antibodies used for staining could shed light on the specificity of the results obtained with this method. Indeed, Cazenave *et al.* (1978) showed that fetal liver cells are very rich in Fc-bearing cells which are able to mediate ADCMC reaction and that this function decreased at birth (Table 2.3).

Furthermore, no alteration in the mitogenic response induced by

TABLE 2.3

Percentage of Cells Bearing Fc Receptors in Fetal and Neonatal Liver and Spleen[a]

Origin of cells	Fetus				Newborn (1 day old)	Neonatal (5 days old)	Adult (12 months old)
	17-day	22-day	26-day	29-day			
Liver	4[b]	ND	9.65	17.51	12.05	3.45	7.16
Spleen	ND[c]	ND	ND	ND	9.1	7.16	26.75

[a] From Cazenave *et al.*, 1978.
[b] Percentage of EA-RFC.
[c] Not done.

levan, galactan, *Salmonella tranoroa* LPS, and dextran was observed on the maternally idiotype-suppressed or adult idiotype-suppressed mice. If identical structures are shared by Ig receptors of mature B cells and mitogen and growth receptors of B cell precursors, it is difficult to understand why anti-Id antibodies have a different activity on the products of the same V genes since they promote the maturation of Ig$^-$ cells to Ig-secreting cells and, in the case of Ig$^+$ cells, turn off the synthesis of Ig.

Finally, it appears that the mother during gestation or suckling period should supply the progeny with anti-Id antibodies. However, these anti-Id antibodies cannot be produced by adults, particularly when natural antibodies produced by immunization with environmental antigens show a high level of idiotypes. This is particularly the case of J558 anti-$\alpha(1\rightarrow3)$dextran, T15 and anti-PC, or X24 anti-galactan antibodies. However, 1-day-old mice are able to make J558$^+$ anti-$\alpha(1\rightarrow3)$dextran or X24$^+$ anti-galactan antibodies in spite of any possible supply of anti-Id antibodies by the mother. It, therefore, appears that until new data and adequate experimental approaches are provided, the problem of the expression of V genes on non-Ig structures remains open.

A possible demonstration of the presence of Id determinants in pre-B cells was provided by Kubagawa *et al.* (1979). In this study two heterologous anti-Id sera were raised against two human myeloma proteins belonging to two different IgA subgroups. Bone marrow cells of these two patients have been stained with labeled anti-Ig and anti-Id reagents. Cells which lacked sIg but which were stained with anti-Id antibodies were identified in bone marrow smears, and these cells were scored as pre-B cells. In these patients the cells which bear sIgM, sIgD, and sIgA were costained by anti-Id reagents, whereas only cIg$^+$ plasma cells were stained with only anti-Id reagents.

This study, in which presumed idiotypic determinants were used as phenotypic markers of V genes and which were found on distinct subpopulations of B cells belonging to the same clone, suggests that cIg$^+$ pre-B cells differentiate into sIg$^+$ small lymphocytes and further into cIg$^+$ plasma cells. Furthermore, this evidence suggests that the antibody diversity and function of V genes begins in the early stage of B cell development, namely, in the pre-B cells. However, problems in the absorption of the antisera used in this study dictate some caution in the interpretation of the results.

III. Sequential Activation of *V* Genes*

In his pioneering studies, Silverstein (1977) demonstrated that responses of the lamb to certain antigens, such as viruses, ferritin, azo-
proteins, ovalbumin, and hemocyanin, could be obtained during fetal
life, whereas responses to diphtheria toxoid, O antigen of *Salmonella
typhosa,* and BCG occurred only after 40 days of postnatal life. Ontogenic delays for other specific antibody responses have been reported in other antigenic systems, suggesting that a genetic
mechanism(s) could be responsible for a sequential activation of *V*
genes.

Immune responses to T-independent antigens represent the best
models to study sequential activation of *V* genes in mice since these
responses are due to direct interactions of antigen with Ig receptors of
precursors of B cells. Therefore, the expression of B cells does not
require helper T cells which themselves mature after birth.

The T-dependent antibody responses require two signals: one produced by antigen and the second by T cells. The delayed onset of the
T-dependent immune responses after birth is often attributed to the
absence of mature T cells (Spear *et al.,* 1973; Hardy *et al.,* 1973;
Spear and Edelman, 1974). Bossing-Schneider (1979) has shown that
only T cells from 9- to 10-day-old mice can produce a replacing factor
which is considered as a second helper factor signal necessary for the
activation of anti-SRBC, a T-dependent antibody response. Haines *et
al.* (1980) have shown that neonatal thymic cells are capable of helping
a direct PFC response but that the switch to an indirect PFC response
is a separate maturation event that occurs between birth and 2 to 4
days of age.

The study of the ontogeny of the immune responses to polysaccharide antigens in BALB/c mice has the advantage that in this strain there
are several myeloma proteins which are specific for various bacteria
polysaccharides (Potter, 1977). Anti-polysaccharide antibodies share
the idiotypes of myeloma proteins specific for levan, inulin, galactan,
lipopolysaccharide.

---

*These data were presented at the 1st Gunsberg Symposium on Reproductive
Immunology held at Mount Sinai Medical Center, June, 1980.

1. X24IdX$^+$ Anti-galactan Response

Anti-galactan antibodies produced by BALB/c mice in response to immunization with gum ghatti share X24IdI and IdX of XRPC24 galactan-binding myeloma protein (Mushinski and Potter, 1977). The anti-galactan response is T-dependent (C. Bona *et al.*, unpublished data). One-day-old BALB/c mice immunized with gum ghatti developed a significant anti-galactan PFC response and about 30% of the anti-galactan PFC secreted X24IdX$^+$ antibodies (Fig. 2.1).

The X24IdX and X24IdI anti-galactan antibodies have been detected in the sera of 1-day-old BALB/c mice immunized with gum ghatti. Therefore, these results indicate that the precursor of anti-galactan antibody-forming cells can be activated after birth.

2. 384Id$^+$ Anti-LPS Response

MOPC384 myeloma protein binds specifically d-methyl-D-galactoside, which represents the immuno-dominant sugar of *Salmonella tranoroa, S. tel-aviv,* and *Proteus mirabilis* LPS. We have found that the 384Id is expressed only on a small fraction of anti-LPS antibodies produced by BALB/c mice. Furthermore, we have observed that 1-day-old BALB/c mice immunized with 10 μg *S. tranoroa* LPS were able to make anti-LPS which expressed the 384Id (Table 2.4).

3. Anti-$\beta(2\rightarrow6)$fructosan Antibody Response

$\beta(2\rightarrow6)$Fructosan antigenic determinant is borne by grass levan and bacterial levan produced by *A. laevanicum, Bacillus subtilis,* and *C. laevanicum.* Bacterial levan (BL) is constituted by a backbone represented by $\beta(2\rightarrow6)$fructosan with $\beta(2\rightarrow1)$ branch points. BALB/c mice immunized with BL produce antibodies of two types. One group of molecules is specific for inulin (Inu), which is a $\beta(2\rightarrow1)$polyfructosan, as well as for levan. The majority of these antibodies expressed idiotypes of inulin-binding myeloma proteins. The second family of antibodies is specific only for $\beta(2\rightarrow6)$fructosan and fails to express the IdX borne by Inu-binding myeloma protein (Bona *et al.*, 1978).

Surprisingly, only anti-BL antibodies which do not cross-react with inulin and do not express IdX can be detected in 1-day-old BALB/c mice in response to immunization with BL (Table 2.4).

This anti-$\beta(2\rightarrow6)$fructosan antibody response seems to be under the control of *Xid* gene, since (CBA/N × BALB/c)F$_1$ males and

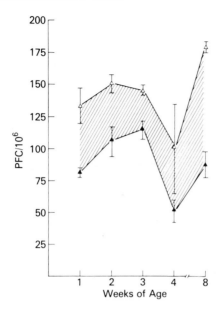

Fig. 2.1. PFC response to gum ghatti 7 days after immunization of BALB/c mice at different ages. Each point represents the mean of 10 mice. △—△, total galactan PFC; △—△, anti-galactan PFC noninhibited by A/He anti-X24Id serum diluted 1:300 and added to agarose; hatched area between curves: X24 Id⁺ fraction.

backcross defective (CBA/N × C3H/HeJ) × C₃H/HeJ males which have an X-linked genetic defect of the maturation of B cells cannot make anti-BL antibodies (Paul *et al.*, 1979; Bona *et al.*, 1980a).

These data show that the precursors of anti-galactan, anti-levan, and anti-LPS can be activated immediately after birth by the corresponding antigens.

4. 460-Id⁺ Anti-TNP Response

MOPC460 myeloma protein binds DNP and TNP haptens. The 460Id cannot be detected in the sera of nonimmunized BALB/c or allotypic congenic BALB/c mice with monoclonal or syngeneic anti-460Id antibodies (Bona *et al.*, 1978). However, after the immunization with T-independent (Bona *et al.*, 1979a) or T-dependent (Zeldis *et al.*, 1979) TNP conjugates the BALB/c mice develop a 460-Id⁺ anti-TNP response.

We have studied recently the ontogeny of the expression of 460Id

TABLE 2.4

Early Occurrence of the Anti-bacterial Levan (BL), *Salmonella tranoroa* Lipopolysaccharide (LPS) and Galactan Antibody Responses

Age of BALB/c mice	Immunization	HA titer (ln units) (BL)	HI titer (E109IdX)	PFC response (10^6) BL	E109[+] (%)
A. Ontogeny of the anti-BL response					
1 day old	Nil	0.3 ± 0.3	0	5 ± 2	0
1 day old[a]	10 μg BL	1.8 ± 0.4	0	46 ± 7	0
9 days old	Nil	2.0 ± 0.3	0	14 ± 7	0
9 days old[a]	10 μg BL	5.1 ± 0.8	0	89 ± 13	0
8 weeks old	Nil	3.8 ± 0.4	1.2 ± 0.4	21 ± 5	32
8 weeks old[a]	10 μg BL	9.5 ± 0.9	3.9 ± 0.5	156 ± 25	43

Age of BALB/c mice	Immunization	HA titer (ln units) (SRBC-LPS)	HI titer (ln units) 384Id		
B. Ontogeny of the anti-LPS response					
1 day old	Nil	1.2 ± 0.3	0		
1 day old[b]	10 μg LPS	4.1 ± 1.8	2.0 ± 0		
8 weeks old	Nil	2.8 ± 0.5	1.2 ± 0.3		
8 weeks old[b]	10 μg LPS	8.7 ± 1.2	4.4 ± 0.5		

Age of BALB/c mice	anti-GAL PFC response (%x24Id[+])	RIA[c] dilution of serum giving 50% inhibition X24IdI	X24IdX
C. Ontogeny of the anti-galactan response			
1 day old	130 ± 24	44	0.052	0.025
7 days old	150 ± 12	42	0.059	0.0255
14 days old	148 ± 12	30	0.105	0.044
21 days old	115 ± 42	51	0.0254	0.039

[a] Anti-BL response was tested 5 days after immunization.
[b] Anti-LPS response was tested 5 days after immunization.
[c] RIA, radioimmunoassay.

on the anti-TNP antibody response. Seven-day-old BALB/c mice immunized with TNP-LPS and TNP-BL produced anti-TNP antibodies which express 460Id. An anti-TNP response was observed only in 2-week-old BALB/c mice after the immunization with TNP-Ficoll. The anti-TNP antibodies produced by 4-week-old mice in response to immunization with TNP-Ficoll express 460Id.

These data indicate that 460Id is expressed very early after immunization with TI-1 T-independent TNP conjugate and later during postnatal life after immunization with TI-2 T-independent conjugates (C. Bona *et al.,* unpublished results) (Table 2.5).

5. T15+ Anti-phosphocholine (PC) Antibody Response

The Id determinants of T15, PC-binding myeloma proteins are found on more than 30% of anti-PC antibodies produced by BALB/c mice in response to immunization with R36A pneumococcal vaccine.

TABLE 2.5

Ontogeny of the Response of BALB/c Mice to Bacterial Levan and Inulin Coupled to T-Dependent and T-Independent Carriers[a]

Age of animals (weeks)	Immunogen	Anti-inulin PFC/10⁶ spleen cells		Anti-inulin titer (HA) (ln)	E109 idiotype titer (HI) (ln)
		Total	% E109+		
2	*Aerobacter* BL	0	0	1	0
	subtilis BL	1 ± 1			
	BL-BA	16 ± 3	2.5 ± 2.5	−1	0
	BL-SRBC[b]	0	0	ND[c]	ND
	Inulin-BA	5 ± 1	0	0	0
8	*Aerobacter* BL	63 ± 1	30 ± 6	8	7
	subtilis BL	130 ± 15	65 ± 3	10	3
	BL-BA	104 ± 12	35 ± 12	7	7
	BL-SRBC[b]	16 ± 4	100 ±	ND	ND
	Inulin-BA	35 ± 6	86 ± 12	8	9

[a] Mice of 2 or 8 weeks of age were immunized with BL (10 μg) derived from *Aerobacter levanicum* or *Bacillus subtilis*, with 0.1 ml of a 1% suspension of BL-BA or inulin-BA or with 0.1 ml of a 10% suspension of BL-SRBC. Their anti-inulin splenic PFC responses and serum anti-inulin HA titers and serum E109 HI titers were determined 5 days later.

[b] PFC were tested on inulin-Burro RBC.

[c] ND, not done.

Signal *et al.* (1976) developed a method to determine the frequency of B cells responsive to PC, namely, an *in vitro* splenic focus technique. The majority of PC-specific precursor cells in adult BALB/c mice are of single T15 clonotype. They found that the PC-responsive cells appear relatively late in neonatal period and can be detected only 4–5 days after birth. Similar results were obtained by Fung *et al.* (1980). These data indicated that neonatal B cells behave similarly to adult B cells and that PC-specific B cells are extremely rare in early neonatal spleen cells.

6. IdX Bearing Anti-arsonate (Ars) Antibody Response

Nutt *et al.* (1979) reported data which indicate that B cells expressing IdX associated with anti-Ars antibodies of mice bearing *Ig-1^c* allotype are present in neonatal mice. One-day-old A/J and CAL20 mice immunized with KHL-Ars conjugates and bled on day 21 made IdX-bearing anti-Ars antibodies. The level of IdX was comparable to that determined in adults. Similar results were obtained when spleen cells from 1-day-old CAL20 were transferred to 400-rad pretreated BALB/c adult mice. (CAL20 mice are congenic with BALB/c and have *Igh-V^c* and *Igh-C^c* genes.) The recipient BALB/c mice were immunized 1 day after the infusion of CAL20 cells, and the response was tested by 21 days. The concentration of IdX in the recipient BALB/c infused with 1-day-old or adult CAL20 spleen cells was similar. Although in these experiments the bleedings were carried out at day 21, it seems that the precursors of IdX$^+$ anti-Ars antibody-forming cells were present before day 7 in the life of the mice. Even in adult mice the level of IdX-bearing anti-Ars antibody is not measurable until 14 days after immunization. With a view to establish more precisely the occurrence of the precursors, the authors took advantage of their previous observation of B cell dominance, i.e., inhibition by BALB/c primed cells (i.e., by a carrier-Ars conjugate) of the expression of IdX-bearing anti-Ars antibodies in CAL20 mice. The results of this type of experiment indicated that B cells bearing IdX$^+$ anti-Ars receptors should be present before day 9 of the neonatal period in CAL20 mice. These results suggested that the IdX anti-Ars response appears at about the same time as the T15 and anti-Pc response in mice.

7. IdX$^+$ Anti-$\beta(2\rightarrow1)$fructosan (Inulin) Response

The study of the ability to produce anti-inulin antibodies and cross-reactive idiotypes in BALB/c mice indicated that it appears late in ontogeny (Bona *et al.*, 1979d). Similar results were obtained by studying the presence of anti-inulin antibody by hemagglutination, PFC (Fig. 2.2), and isoelectric focusing assays. A weak anti-inulin PFC response was observed in 21-day-old BALB/c mice, a substantial increase at 28 days, and PFC-secreting anti-inulin antibodies bearing IdX have been found by 60 days of age. In view of the failure of young BALB/c mice to make anti-inulin antibodies in response to immunization with bacterial levan (BL), we studied whether the presentation of inulin or BL on carriers that are known to stimulate the B cells might elicit the production of anti-inulin antibodies. Inulin and levan conjugated with SRBC or *Brucella abortus*, which are active carriers in young animals, were used in an attempt to stimulate early occurrence of the anti-inulin response. Both were ineffective in stimulating inulin-specific B cells (Table 2.6). The B cell polyclonal activators could discern the precursor in very young stages and even in suppressed states (Trenkner and Riblet, 1975; Fernandez *et al.*, 1979; Bona *et al.*, 1977). We have studied the occurrence of anti-inulin PFC after the *in vitro* stimulation of young cells with NWSM. Upon stimulation with NWSM a significant [^{3}H]thymidine incorporation was observed by spleen cells from 1-week-old animals. By contrast, an anti-inulin response was not detected until the donors were 4 weeks of age. These results have indicated that the inability of young mice to make anti-inulin antibody was secondary to the absence or lack of maturity of the precursor of anti-inulin antibody-forming cells (Fig. 2.3). With a view to study whether the unresponsiveness of young mice to immunization with inulin-BA might be due to the immaturity of accessory cells, we studied the anti-inulin response in CB20 mice. CB20 mice possess the same H-2 background as BALB/c mice but have *Igh-V* and *Igh-C* genes of C57BL/Ka mice and therefore are not able to develop an IdX$^+$ anti-inulin response. We reconstituted 300-rad CB20 mice with spleen cells from 1-week-old BALB/c mice, and immediately the mice were immunized with inulin-BA. No anti-inulin antibody or E109$^+$ molecules were detected. By contrast, if the immunization of the recipients injected with 1-week-old BALB/c was delayed until 7 or 14 days after cell transfer, a significant E109IdX$^+$ anti-inulin antibody

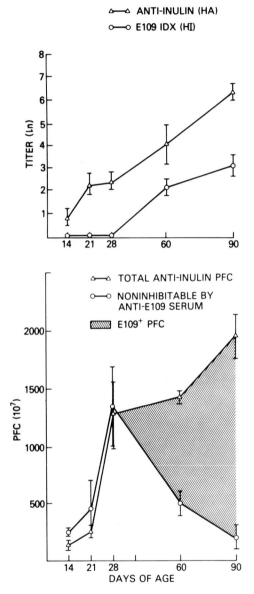

Fig. 2.2. Age dependence of anti-inulin response of BALB/c mice. (*Top*) Serum antibody response 5 days after immunization of BALB/c of various ages with bacterial levan (BL) (10 μg). (*Bottom*) Anti-inulin PFC response 5 days after immunization of BALB/c of various ages with BL (10 μg).

TABLE 2.6

Anti-inulin Response of C.B20 Recipients of Spleen Cells BALB/c mice[a,b]

	Time of immunization[c]	No. mice tested	Anti-inulin PFC/10⁶ cells		Anti-inulin titer (HA) (ln)	E109 IdX titer (HI) (ln)
			Total	% E109⁺		
BALB/c adult mice	—[d]	3	260 ± 108	51 ± 22	4 ± 1	5 ± 1
C.B20 adult mice	—	3	35 ± 14	3 ± 3	2 ± 1	0
Irradiated C.B20 mice	0	3	17 ± 14	8 ± 8	1 ± 1	0
Irradiated C.B20 mice given 1-week-old BALB/c cells	0	6	7 ± 5	4 ± 4	0.5 ± 0.5	0
	7	3	80 ± 50	20 ± 12	3 ± 2	0
	14	3	75 ± 49	36 ± 17	3 ± 1	1.3 ± 0.3
Irradiated C.B20 mice given 3-week-old BALB/c cells	0	3	83 ± 4	35 ± 12	2 ± 0.5	2 ± 1
Irradiated C.B20 mice given 8-week-old BALB/c cells	0	6	119 ± 13	54 ± 14	3 ± 1	3 ± 1

[a] From Bona et al., 1979d.

[b] 5×10^7 Spleen cells from 1-, 3-, and 8-week-old mice.

[c] Adult C.B20 mice received 300 R of X irradiation and then received 5×10^7 spleen cells from 1-, 3-, or 8-week-old BALB/c mice. They were immunized with 0.1 ml of a 1% suspension of inulin-BA either on the day of transfer (day 0) or 7 or 14 days after transfer.

[d] As controls, nonirradiated adult BALB/c and C.B20 mice were immunized. Anti-inulin splenic PFC, serum anti-inulin HA titers, and serum E109 IdX titers were measured 7 days after immunization.

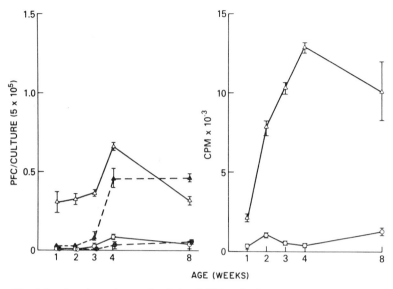

Fig. 2.3. Age dependence of polyclonal PFC and mitogenic responses. Left: 5 × 10⁵ spleen cells from BALB/c mice of various ages were stimulated for 3 days with 10 μg NWSM. ○, anti-BL PFC in control cultures; △, in cultures stimulated with NWSM. ●, anti-inulin PFC in control cultures; and ▲ in cultures stimulated with NWSM. Right; uptake of [³H]thymidine by 2 × 10⁵ spleen cells from BALB/c of various ages stimulated for 3 days with 30 μg of NWSM. ○, control cultures; △, cultures stimulated with NWSM. From Bona *et al.*, 1979b.

response was observed. These results indicate that unresponsiveness of 1-week-old BALB/c mice was not related to the absence of environmental antigens or immaturity of accessory cells (Table 2.7). Furthermore, this unresponsiveness was not linked to the presence of suppressor cells in young animals, since the infusion of young T cells into adult BALB/c animal did not affect IdX⁺ anti-inulin response, whereas BALB/c adult cells infused in 1-week-old BALB/c were able to respond to immunization with inulin-BA (Table 2.8). The data presented above indicate that the capacity of BALB/c mice to make anti-inulin antibodies and to express two of the principal anti-inulin IdX determinants (G and B) is not acquired until 4 weeks of age and reflects a delay in the appearance of the anti-inulin precursor cells rather than either a lack of immunogenicity of the antigen in young mice or the existence of an active mechanism preventing the response (Bona *et al.*, 1979d).

TABLE 2.7

Lack of Evidence of Suppression of Anti-inulin Response in Young Animals[a]

Mice[b]	Anti-inulin PFC/10^6 cells		HA titer (ln)		HI titer (ln)	
	Total	% E109+	BL	Inulin	IdX-G	IdX-A
A. Adult BALB/c mice irradiated with 200 R and infused with						
Control[c]	130 ± 29	24 ± 6	4 ± 1	4 ± 0	4 ± 0	4 ± 0
3 × 10^7 adult BALB/c T-cells	72 ± 16	18 ± 3	4 ± 0	4 ± 0	4 ± 0	2 ± 1
3 × 10^7 2-week-old BALB/c T-cells	166 ± 10	32 ± 6	6 ± 1	5 ± 1	4 ± 0	4 ± 1
B. 1-week-old BALB/c mice infused with						
Control[c]	4 ± 4	6 ± 5	3.7 ± 0.3	0.7 ± 0.5	0	2 ± 0
5 × 10^7 1-week-old BALB/c spleen cells	3 ± 2	0	2.5 ± 0.3	1.8 ± 0.2	0.3 ± 0.3	1.5 ± 0.5
5 × 10^7 adult BALB/c spleen cells	33 ± 7	30 ± 9	6 ± 0.7	2.8 ± 0.2	4.2 ± 0.2	2.5 ± 0.3

[a] From Bona et al., 1979d.
[b] Four mice in each group; mice were immunized with 10 μg BL and the response was studied 5 days after immunization.
[c] Not infused with cells.

TABLE 2.8

Ontogeny of Anti-BL and Anti-inulin Antibody and of Expression of IdX[a]

Age of BALB/c mice (days)	Immunization with 10 μg BL	HA titer (ln)		HI titer (ln)		
		BL	Inulin	IdXG	IdXB	IdXA
7	−	1	0	0	0	1
	+	3	0	0	0	1
14	−	1	1	0	0	3
	+	3	1	0	0	4
21	−	3	1	0	1	3
	+	7	1	0	3	5
28	−	2	2	0	2	2
	+	8	3	3	7	6
84	−	3	4	2	6	2
	+	12	8	5	11	8

[a] Groups of five BALB/c mice of the ages indicated were immunized with BL or were not immunized. The mice were bled 5 days later, and the sera were pooled and tested for anti-BL and anti-inulin hemagglutinin and for IdX-G, -B, and -A.

9. Anti-α(1→6)dextran Response

Howard and Hale in 1976 reported that the anti-α(1→6) dextran antibody response occurred particularly late in mice. Fernandez and Moller (1978) studied more extensively the causes of this delayed antibody response. They concluded that the Ig+ precursor of anti-α(1→6)dextran antibody-forming cells do not exist in 1-month-old mice, whereas cells bearing mitogen receptors for dextran can be observed. At 55 days of age the anti-α(1→6)dextran response represented only 10% of that of mice 3 months of age. These authors have also clearly shown that this late response was not related to the existence of suppressor cells.

The late occurrence of certain anti-polysaccharide T-independent antibody responses reviewed above cannot be ascribed to lack of *V* genes which encode the IdXs of these late responses. Actually the animals later were able to respond to these antigens and to mount an IdX positive response.

It seems unlikely that this late maturation of the response can be explained by a "tolerance state" of the precursors in the young animals. In the case of late anti-β(2→1)fructosan response, the tolerogen would have to be inulin-like rather than BL-like since lack of responsiveness was limited only to $\beta(2\rightarrow1)$fructosan epitopes and not to $\beta(2\rightarrow6)$ epitopes, both of which are carried by bacterial levan. Obviously, there is no source of inulin in the neonatal flora. Additionally, the experimental tolerance requires 1 mg of BL, and such a concentration does not seem likely to be achieved by the antigen supplied via the placenta or milk from the mother.

Finally in the case of anti-$\beta(2\rightarrow1)$fructosan and anti-α-$(1\rightarrow6)$dextran responses, the B cell mitogen were not able to activate the precursors of anti-$\beta(2\rightarrow1)$fructosan and anti-$\alpha(1\rightarrow6)$dextran despite the fact that other subsets of B cells in 1- to 4-week old mice have been stimulated polyclonally by bacterial levan and dextran. Another explanation of this late maturation of some *V* genes can be related to the fact that the stimulation of virgin B cells may be highly affinity dependent (Klinman, 1972). However, Siskind (1979) has shown that B cells from fetal liver already have antigen receptors of both high and low affinity and that their ability to respond to antigens matures with time. This sequential activation of *V* genes suggests that the adult B clonotype immune repertoire is acquired by antigen-independent generative events and that a particular genetic mechanism(s) determines the time when a particular *V* gene is activated. Several explanations that we discussed at the 1st International Gunsberg Symposium on Reproductive Immunology can be entertained to explain the sequential activation of *V* genes as follows:

a. Existence of a genetic mechanism which regulates a random activation of *V* genes in which the regulatory genes can play an important role.

b. An order of activation of *V* genes which could correspond to a translation of *V* genes forth from *C* genes. Accordingly, the *V*–*C* translocation continues during postnatal life and the combinatorial joining of *V* genes begins with the *V* genes nearest to the *J* and *C* genes and sequentially progress to more distal *V* genes. By a sequential loop and excision mechanism all *V* genes would be brought into position for transcription of B clones.

c. The sequential activation can be related to a programmed mutational process which would permit an adult to express a large number of antibody specificities from a limited pool of information, as was emphasized by Klinman *et al.* (1976). In this case new genes coding for new Id specificities could derive from a common ancestor. A candidate of a common ancestor which occurred early in ontogeny and from which IdX$^+$ (B,G) anti-inulin antibody-forming cells might be derived has been found in the anti-inulin antibody response. Indeed, in the serum of immunized and nonimmunized 1- and 2-week-old BALB/c mice we have detected IdXA$^+$ molecules (Table 2.8). These IdXA$^+$ molecules have not been removed with both inulin- or levan-coated SRBC, indicating that IdXA was not associated with high-affinity antibodies. By contrast IdXG -B and -A anti-inulin antibodies produced by adult animals have been removed by this adsorption procedure (Bona *et al.*, 1979c). The precursors of such IdXA$^+$-secreting cells are interesting candidates for antecedents of IdXG$^+$-A$^+$-B$^+$ bearing anti-inulin antibody-forming cells of older BALB/c mice. Thus, the mechanism responsible for sequential activation of V-*h* genes can account for some aspects of diversification of antibodies.

IV. Maternal Idiotype Suppression

Maternal idiotype suppression has as its basic principle the suppression of the father's idiotype in F$_1$ hybrids by immunization of the mothers against the father's idiotype. Maternal idiotype suppression was first studied by Weiler *et al.* (1977) in the $\alpha(1\rightarrow3)$dextran system in which the J558 IdX$^+$ anti-$\alpha(1\rightarrow3)$dextran response occurs early in the ontogeny. They obtained idiotype-suppressed F$_1$ hybrids by mating BALB/c males with SJL females previously immunized with J558 myeloma protein of BALB/c origin. Of 112 progeny tested, 111 were fully suppressed up to 12 weeks of age. A release from the suppression was observed at 20 weeks of age. However, half of the mice which escaped from the suppression did not express J558 IdX on anti-$\alpha(1\rightarrow3)$dextran antibodies in response to the immunization with B1355 dextran. In the J558 Id-suppressed mice the anti-phosphocholine response was completely normal, indicating that the suppression was limited to the anti-$\alpha(1\rightarrow3)$dextran clones.

Similarly, in the levan–inulin system we succeeded in inducing a specific maternal idiotype suppression (Bona *et al.*, 1979b). Female CB20 mice were immunized with E109 myeloma protein prior to mating with BALB/c male (E109 is an inulin-binding myeloma protein of BALB/c origin). The progeny of this mating were immunized with bacterial levan at 4 months of age. Their response was compared to those of normal (CB20 × BALB/c)F_1 and to F_1 progeny originating from a cross of CB20 immunized with XRPC-24 (i.e., a galactan-binding myeloma protein) and then mated with BALB/c. The anti-inulin response of F_1 hybrids was completely suppressed when they originated from CB20 immunized with E109 myeloma protein. This suppression was assessed by HA, IEF, and PFC assay (Table 2.9 and Fig. 2.4). Although no IdXG^+ and B^+ anti-inulin antibodies have been detected in these mice, we found in their sera IdXA^+ molecules. This observation is quite in keeping with our previous results that IdXA^+ molecules devoid of anti-inulin activity were found in 2-week-old mice. It is not clear why the clone secreting IdXA^+ molecules was not susceptible to suppression. This clone could represent an entirely independent line of precursors that merely bears an idiotype cross-reactive with that of anti-inulin antibodies.

The maternal idiotype suppression was also obtained in F_1 and BALB/c hybrids originating from BALB/c mice immunized against their self-idiotypes. Since all normal BALB/c mice express small titers to dextran or phosphocholine because of natural stimulation by environmental antigens, BALB/c cannot be used normally for a maternal idiotype suppression type of experiment. However, Cosenza *et al.* (1977) obtained maternal idiotype suppression in BALB/c hybrids by using BALB/c female animals suppressed after birth with A/J anti-T15IdX antibodies. These neonatal suppressed females were immunized with TEPC15 myeloma protein at maturation and then were mated with BALB/c males. All the offspring tested were completely suppressed at 7 and 10 weeks of age. Similar results were obtained with BALB/c mice immunized against J558 myeloma protein and then mated with BALB/c. Eight out of 13 F_1 hybrids did not express J558 IdX. However, Weiler (1981) considered that hybrid (SLJ × BALB/c) mothers were much more effective than BALB/c mothers in suppressing the J558IdX anti-dextran antibody response.

It was assumed after the discovery of allotype suppression in rabbits that IgG which can cross the placental barrier is responsible for the maternal effect. In an elegant experiment Weiler *et al.* (1977) clearly showed that more than transplacental transmission of anti-Id antibodies is responsible for maternal idiotypic suppression. The progeny from mothers immunized with J558 myeloma protein were given half to anti-idiotype mothers and half to normal SJL mothers, and vice

TABLE 2.9

Anti-inulin Response and Serum IdXs in 4-Month-Old Maternally Suppressed (C.B20 × BALB/c)F$_1$ Mice[a,b]

Mice (No.)	Anti-inulin PFC per 10^6 spleen cells			Serum titer (ln)			
	Total	% IdX-G$^+$	% IdX-A$^+$	Anti-inulin HA	IdX-G HI	IdX-A HI
(C.B20 × BALB/c)F$_1$ (7)	43 ± 12	50	70	3 ± 0	3 ± 0.3	7.3 ± 3
C.B20 anti-E109 × BALB/c)F$_1$ (5)	0	n.d.	n.d.	0	0	5.8 ± 0.4
C.B20 anti-XRPC-24 × BALB/c)F$_1$ (5)	45 ± 12	45	n.d.	3.2 ± 1.1	3.5 ± 0.7	6.8 ± 1.8

[a] From Bona et al., 1979b.

[b] Mice were immunized with 10 μg BL PFC and serum antibody responses were tested 5 days after immunization. IdX-G$^+$ anti-inulin PFC were detected by inhibition as a result of addition of C.B20 anti-E109 antiserum (1:100) to the agarose. IdX-A$^+$ anti-inulin PFC were detected by inhibition with A/He anti-W3082 antiserum.

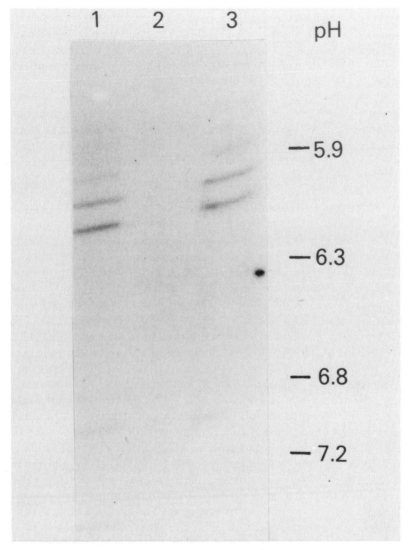

Fig. 2.4. Isoelectric focusing pattern of normal and maternally suppressed (CB20 × BALB/c)F$_1$ mice immunized with 10 μg BL at 4 months of age. (See legend of Fig. 2.2 for details). 1, Normal (CB20 × BALB/c)F$_1$; 2, maternally suppressed (CB20 × BALB/c)F$_1$; 3, normal BALB/c. From Bona *et al.*, 1979d.

versa. All the mice nursed by anti-Id mothers were suppressed, and some of F_1 originating from anti-Id mothers nursed by normal mothers expressed J558 IdX after immunization with dextran. These results clearly showed that the effect of anti-Id antibodies transmitted via milk are as important as placental effects.

It, therefore, appears that the precursor of cells bearing Id^+ Ig receptors can be suppressed by maternal anti-Id antibodies transmitted to progeny via placenta or milk. The transmission via milk explains the possibility of inducing a "maternal" suppression even in the case when the precursors occur late in ontogeny.

V. Neonatal Idiotype Suppression

Neonatal idiotype suppression was obtained in several antigenic systems by administration of heterologous or homologous anti-Id antibodies after birth. Supporting evidence for neonatal idiotype suppression comes from several studies.

Pawlak *et al.* (1973b) induced a long-lasting suppression in A/J mice injected with 1 mg of rabbit anti-IdX Ars antibodies 3 days after birth. At 5 months of age these mice had completely suppressed the IdX^+ component of anti-Ars antibodies while the anti-KLH response was not altered.

Strayer *et al.* (1975) induced neonatal suppression in BALB/c mice injected twice with 0.1 mg A/J anti-T151dX antisera the first week after birth. When these mice were immunized at 2–8 months of age they did not develop a $T151dX^+$ anti-phosphocholine response comparable to control mice. By contrast, suppressed and control mice equally responded to TNP or horse red blood cells. The unresponsiveness was not related to the presentation of antigen since they did not show a normal response after immunization with phosphocholine T-dependent or T-independent antigens. The neonatal suppression was a long-term suppression compared to short-term suppression obtained in adults and was not broken by *in vitro* culture of cells from suppressed animals.

Kohler (1975) did not find cells stained with fluoresceinated anti-T15 antibodies in the 4- or 24-hour cultures of cells from neonatal suppressed mice. By contrast, after 4 hours of culture of cells from adult suppressed mice, the number of cells stained was equal to those of normal mice.

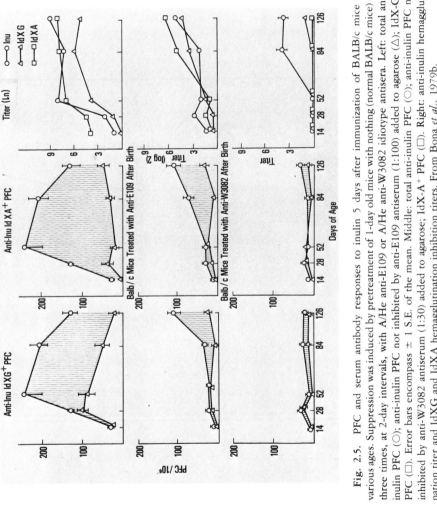

Fig. 2.5. PFC and serum antibody responses to inulin 5 days after immunization of BALB/c mice of various ages. Suppression was induced by pretreatment of 1-day old mice with nothing (normal BALB/c mice) or three times, at 2-day intervals, with A/He anti-E109 or A/He anti-W3082 idiotype antisera. Left: total anti-inulin PFC (○); anti-inulin PFC not inhibited by anti-E109 antiserum (1:100) added to agarose (△); IdX-G⁺ PFC (□). Middle: total anti-inulin PFC (○); anti-inulin PFC not inhibited by anti-W3082 antiserum (1:30) added to agarose; IdX-A⁺ PFC (□). **Right:** anti-inulin hemagglutination titer and IdXG and IdXA hemagglutination inhibition titers. From Bona *et al.*, 1979b.

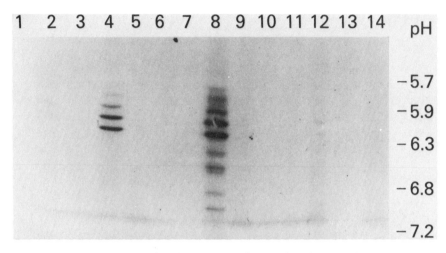

Fig. 2.6. Isoelectric focusing pattern of normal and neonatally suppressed BALB/c mice immunized with 10 μg bacterial levan (BL) at various ages. (See legend of Fig. 2.2 for details.) Normal BALB/c mice immunized with BL at age: 1, 1 week; 2, 2 weeks; 3, 3 weeks; 4, 12 weeks. BALB/c mice pretreated at 1, 3, and 5 days of age with A/He anti-E109 idiotype antiserum and immunized with BL at age: 5, 1 week; 6, 2 weeks; 7, 3 weeks; 8, 12 weeks. BALB/c mice pretreated at 1, 3, and 5 days of age with A/He anti-W3082 idiotype antiserum and immunized with BL at age: 9, 1 week; 10, 2 weeks; 11, 3 weeks; 12, 4 weeks; 13, 6 weeks 14, 16 weeks. From Bona *et al.,* 1979b.

Augustin and Cosenza (1976) observed that during neonatal-induced idiotypic suppression the T15[+] is dominant and more than 90% of anti-phosphocholine antibodies express this IdX. This observation indicates that the interplay between idiotype and anti-idiotype during early life can dramatically change the pattern of response and can lead to the expression of clones which belong to the silent repertoire.

Neonatal idiotype suppression was also obtained in the levan–inulin antigenic system by injection of 1-day-old BALB/c mice with A/He anti-E109 or anti-W3082Id antibodies (Bona *et al.,* 1979b). E109 is an IdXG[+] -A[+] -B[−] and W3082 is an IdXG[+] A[+] -B[+] inulin-binding myeloma protein. Animals treated as neonates with anti-E109Id antibodies did not exhibit IdXA[+] and G[+] anti-inulin PFC until 80 days of age. Suppression induced with anti-W3802Id antibodies was even longer (Figs. 2.5 and 2.6).

The results indicating that maternal and neonatal suppression of the

T15$^+$ anti-PC and IdXG$^+$ -A$^+$ anti-inulin responses can be quite easily induced is at first somewhat surprising in view of the ontogenic delay of both responses. Two explanations can be entertained: (a) precursors of anti-PC and anti-inulin may be present in neonates and although not competent to respond to inulin and phosphocholine may be susceptible to suppression. (b) The maternally transferred or neonatally injected antibodies may persist until the appearance of IdX$^+$ precursors and then suppress them. In any event, the maternal and neonatal idiotypic suppression indicates that the precursors of antibody-forming cells are particularly susceptible to this type of suppression.

Variation of Idiotypes during the Immune Response

In the poly- or pauciclonal antibody responses, the antigen stimulates several clones which secrete antibodies that can express the same or various idiotypic specificities. In addition, a particular antigen does not necessarily activate the whole complementary specific immune repertoire. Various idiotypic specificities can change during the immune response until the secretion of antibodies begins to decline. In certain immune responses the cyclic pattern can be related to the occurrence of anti-idiotype antibodies which can profoundly alter the pattern of idiotypes by suppression of major idiotypes expressed during earlier stages of the response and which favor the occurrence of new idiotypes which had been silent or had represented a minor fraction of the repertoire.

I. Persistence and Variation of Idiotypes during the Immune Response

Soon after the discovery of the idiotypy in the rabbit, Oudin and Michel (1969b) reported a new observation concerning the variation of idiotypic specificities in a rabbit immunized with *Salmonella typhi* which was bled 37 times during 3 years. Raising adequate anti-idiotypic antisera, Oudin was able to discriminate three idiotypic specificities in a serum sample obtained after the fifth bleeding (S5) and four new idiotypes after the thirty-seventh bleeding (S37). Interestingly, the three early occurring idiotypes were found in both serum samples (S5 and S37) in spite of the 29 month interval between the two bleedings. These results indicated that among the antibodies produced by an individual rabbit following immunization with a particular "O" antigen, the number of idiotypes seemed to increase during the immune response. This observation suggested that several clones which produce various antibodies with the same antigenic specificity are responsible for the heterogeneity of the antibody response. In the antibody response of a rabbit immunized with *Salmonella abortus equi,* Oudin and Bordenave (1971) observed the disappearance of an early expressed idiotype and the occurrence of new idiotypes in the late phase of the immune response.

In the same vein, MacDonald and Nisonoff (1970) observed persistence and changes of idiotypic specificities during the anti-arsonate antibody response in the rabbit. Thus, the idiotypic specificities observed in the second month bleeding (i.e., performed after the last immunization) persisted until 4 months when a drastic change of idiotypic pattern was observed. The idiotypes expressed during the first 4 months disappeared and new idiotypic specificities emerged. In fact, the anti-Id antibodies prepared against the antibodies of the eighth month bleeding interacted with the antibodies of the fifth month bleeding but not with those of the second to fourth month bleedings. The antibodies which expressed the idiotypes of the eighth month bleeding were present for at least 1 year from months 5 to 17.

A recent study performed in humans indicated persistence of the same idiotypic specificity on anti-Rh antibodies of a volunteer during 12 years (between 1968 and 1977). The subject was immunized four times at 3 months intervals in 1968 and 1969 and one time in 1970 and 1972. The rabbit anti-Id antiserum was prepared against anti-Rh antibodies from the 1974 bleeding. This anti-Id antiserum interacted with anti-Rh antibodies produced by this subject during 12 years (de Saint Martin *et al.,* 1978).

In mice we have studied the kinetics of anti-galactan PFC response and the expression of XRPC24IdI and -IdX. Mushinsky and Potter (1977) had shown that IdX and IdI of XRPC24 galactan-binding myeloma protein are expressed on anti-galactan antibodies produced in BALB/c mice following immunization with gum ghatti. The kinetics of the anti-galactan antibody response were studied during a period of 150 days in adult BALB/c mice immunized with 100 μg gum ghatti; the mice were sacrificed at various intervals after immunization. A significant increase of the anti-galactan PFC response which peaked at 5 and 30 days was observed. Even 150 days after immunization the number of anti-galactan PFC was 20-fold higher than in nonimmunized mice. Between 50 and 90% of anti-galactan PFC have been inhibited by A/He anti-XRPC24IdX antibodies indicating that a substantial fraction of cells which secreted anti-galactan antibodies expressed XRPC24IdX (Fig. 3.1). The level of the XRPC24IdI and -IdX was measured in the same mice by RIA. A significant number of molecules bearing XRPC24IdI and -IdX were detected 10 days after immunization (Table 3.1). The discrepancy between the early increase of the anti-galactan PFC response and the late increase of IdX and IdI in the serum can be explained by the delay required for the accumula-

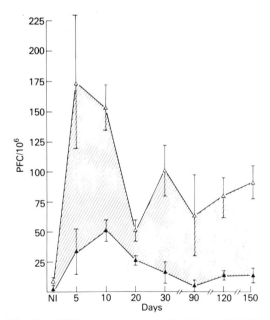

Fig. 3.1. Kinetics of PFC response to gum ghatti in adult BALB/c mice and the fraction of PFC response due to cells secreting X24IdX. $\triangle$————$\triangle$, Anti-galactan PFC. $\blacktriangle$————$\blacktriangle$, anti-galactan PFC in presence of 1:30 A/He anti-X24IdX antibodies; hatched area, PFC X24+. Each points represents the mean of 5 mice. NI indicates the mean of number of PFC in nonimmunized mice.

TABLE 3.1

Kinetics of Serum IdX and IdI after Immunization with Gum Ghatti in Adult BALB/c Mice

Day	No. of mice	RIA (dilution of serum giving 50% inhibition)[a]	
		IdX	IdI
5	5	0.110, 0.129,[b] $<$, $<$, $<$	0.10, 0.091, $<$, $<$, $<$
10	3	0.044, 0.0098, 0.021	$<$, 0.153, 0.020
20	8	0.55, 0.255, $<$, 0.106, $<$, $<$, $<$, 0.1176	$<$, 0,192, $<$, $<$, $<$, $<$, 0.153
30	8	0.0668, 0.0756, 0.086, 0.0976, 0.088, 0.018, 0.0111, 0.0156,	0.172, $<$, $<$, 0.062, 0.31, 0.040 $<$, $<$, 0.062 0.31, 0.040, $<$, $<$
90	3	0.0289, 0.0129, 0.0126	$<$, 0.0112, 0.377
150	3	0.05, 0.02, 0.163	0.146, $<$, $<$

[a] Values for each mouse respectively: $<$, no inhibition at 1:4 dilution, i.e., < 0.25, 1:10 = 0.1, 1:100 = 0.01 1:1000 = 0.001 determined from a regressive curve.
[b] Mice number tested.

tion of the products of antibody-secreting cells in the serum. The proportion of IdX and IdI bearing antigalactan antibodies increased with time, and the great majority of anti-galactan antibodies expressed XRPC24IdI and IdX by 90–150 days.

Monoclonal antibodies represent an invaluable tool for investigating the persistence and the variation of idiotypes during the immune response. Metzger et al. (1980) studied the expression of idiotypes of monoclonal antibodies produced by hybridomas obtained from the fusion of lymphocytes harvested at various intervals after immunization with hen lysozyme. With anti-Id antibodies prepared against hybridomas obtained in the early phase of the response, it was established that Id determinants of "early" hybridomas were not observed on monoclonal antibodies produced by "later" hybridomas. These data taken collectively show that Id determinants expressed during a particular antibody response can persist and can change during the immune response.

II. Inverse Fluctuation between Idiotype-Bearing Antibodies and Spontaneous Occurrence of Anti-idiotypic Antibodies

There are few instances in which it has been clearly shown that the variation of IdX^+ component of the antibody response is related to the occurrence of anti-Id autoantibodies or anti-Id-forming cells. These anti-Id autoantibodies which occur during the immune response for certain antigens are responsible for the decrease of Id^+-bearing antibodies. The occurrence of these anti-Id autoantibodies has been observed in the systems given below.

A. Phosphocholine (PC)

Kluskens and Kohler (1974) studied the expression of T15IdX on anti-PC antibodies produced by BALB/c mice in response to immunization with *Pneumococcus* R36A vaccine. The cell walls of the R36A strain contain PC antigenic determinants. An increased titer of $T15IdX^+$ anti-PC antibodies as well as anti-PC PFC response was observed 1 week after the completion of immunization. By 12 weeks, the appearance of anti-T15 antibodies was observed in the sera of these mice. It appears that these mice developed anti-T15 antibodies against $T15^+$ anti-PC antibodies which were elicited after immunization with R36A pneumococcal vaccine. By 12–18 weeks when these anti-T15 autoantibodies were detected, a relative decrease of anti-PC antibodies was observed. Cosenza (1976) using a more sensitive PFC assay was able to detect anti-T15 PFC autoantibodies earlier after the immunization with R36A pneumococcal vaccine. He studied simultaneously the kinetics of $T15Id^+$ anti-PC PFC and the anti-T15Id PFC in the same mice during the 12 days following immunization. $T15^+$ anti-PC PFC were observed immediately after immunization, and this response peaked by day 5. A decrease of $T15^+$ and anti-PC PFC response was observed between days 6 and 10. Interestingly, at this time the occurrence of anti-T15 Id was observed. Kelsoe and Cerny (1979) confirmed the existence of this inverse fluctuation between Id^+-bearing antibodies and anti-Id cells by studying the kinetics of production of $T15^+$ anti-PC antibodies and the number of cells able to bind TEPC15 myeloma protein resulting from the appearance of receptors with anti-Id specificity. In this study the authors observed three peaks of anti-PC response at days 2, 10–11, and 14 and two peaks of cells which were specific for T15IdX at days 4 and 12. Therefore, these results show that the decrease of anti-PC response after immunization with R36A pneumococcal vaccine was accompanied by an increase of anti-T14 IdX PFC.

B. Levan—Inulin

Similarly we have observed the occurrence of anti-Id PFC in the anti levan–inulin antibody response (Bona *et al.,* 1978). Adult BALB/c mice which have not been immunized with bacterial levan (BL) have a significant titer of anti-levan antibodies (3.8 ± 0.3) and a lower but significant titer of anti-inulin antibodies (1.9 ± 0.2). Bacterial levan is a $\beta(2{\rightarrow}6)$polyfructosan with $\beta(2{\rightarrow}1)$ branch points, whereas inulin is a $\beta(2{\rightarrow}1)$polyfructosan. The anti-inulin antibodies and a fraction of anti-levan antibodies produced after immunization with BL share the IdXs (G, B, and A) of inulin-binding myeloma proteins (Lieberman *et al.,* 1975). These IdXs are expressed on anti-levan and anti-inulin antibodies found in nonimmunized BALB/c mice. Upon immunization with 10 μg BL, the hemagglutination (HA) titer to levan rises and reaches a peak at 5 to 10 days, falls off slightly, and peaks again at 30 days. The anti-inulin antibodies and IdX titer parallel the cyclic pattern of anti-levan response (Fig. 3.2). The study of the anti-levan and anti-inulin PFC response to 10 μg BL yields a similar time course to that found with hemagglutinins. After immunization, the number of anti-levan and anti-inulin PFC increases rapidly, peaks at day 10, declines, and then reaches a second peak at day 30 (Fig. 3.3). Interestingly, in the very early (5 day) and late (60 day) periods, the majority of anti-inulin PFC were E109IdX-positive, whereas between 10 and 30 days the proportion of both anti-inulin and antilevan PFC was lower. The decline of IdX$^+$ component of anti-levan and anti-inulin response between 10 and 30 days coincided with the occurrence of a small number of anti-E109IdXPFC autoantibodies. This kind of anti-Id PFC autoantibody cannot be detected in normal (nonimmunized) BALB/c mice. These anti-E109-PFC autoantibodies appear to be specific in that they are inhibited with E109 myeloma protein but not by equal concentrations of two non-inulin-binding IgA$_k$ myeloma proteins: ABPC48 which binds $\beta(2{\rightarrow}6)$fructosan and MOPC 167 which binds PC (Table 3.2).

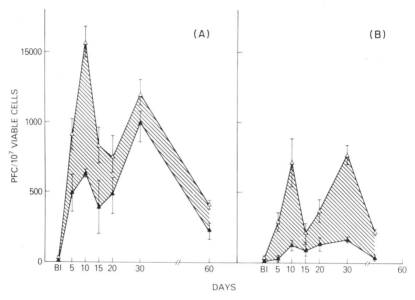

Fig. 3.2. Kinetics of PFC response to levan in adult BALB/c mice and the fraction of the plaque-forming response due to cells secreting the E109 idiotype. A: △————△ anti-levan PFC; ▲————▲, anti-levan PFC in presence of 1:100 anti-E109 serum. B: ▲————▲, anti-inulin PFC in presence of 1:100 anti-E109 serum. Hatched area, E109 positive PFC. Each point represents the mean of six animals except at day 5 where each point represents the mean of twelve animals. BI indicates the mean of number of plaques in nonimmunized mice.

C. TNP

In BALB/c and AKR mice, Goidl *et al.* (1979) observed a decline of the anti-TNP PFC response between 4 and 7 days after immunization. They attributed this decline to putative anti-Id autoantibodies which were bound on the surface of anti-TNP antibody-secreting cells. However, no information was provided in this study concerning the idiotype against which the putative anti-Id antibodies were directed as well as the variation of the level of Id-bearing molecules during the period in which anti-Id antibodies were detected.

D. *Micrococcus lysoleikticus* Polysaccharide

Brown and Rodkey (1979) have reported the appearance of anti-Id autoantibodies in a rabbit immunized three times during a 31-month period with *Micrococcus* polysaccharide. Only anti-polysaccharide antibodies were observed after the first and third immunizations, and the anti-Id autoantibodies were identified after the second immunization. The isoelectric focusing (IEF) analysis of this response provided very interesting data. After the first immunization, several clonotypes which bound the labeled antigen were observed, indicating that this

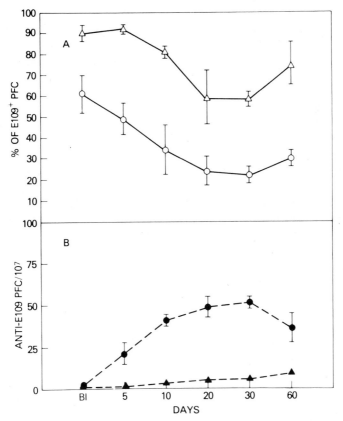

Fig. 3.3. The relationship between anti-levan and anti-inulin PFC carrying E109 idiotype and the number of anti-E109 plaque-forming cells. (A) Percentage of anti-levan and anti-inulin plaque-forming cells carrying the E109 idiotype at various times after immunization with 10 μg levan. ○————○, E109⁺ anti-levan + PFC; △————△, E109⁺ anti-inulin + PFC. (B) The number of anti-E109 plaque-forming cells at various times after immunization with 10 μg levan. ●— — —●, Anti-E109 direct PFC; ▲— — —▲, anti-E109 indirect PFC.

TABLE 3.2

Specificity of Anti-E109 Plaque-Forming Assay[a]

Inhibitor added in plaque-forming assay	Concentration of inhibitor (μg/ml)			
	0	1	10	100
E109 myeloma protein	59 ± 0.5[b]	61 ± 5	37 ± 4	8 ± 3
A48 myeloma protein[c]		58 ± 4	61 ± 11	52 ± 7
MOPC167 myeloma protein[d]		51 ± 3	36 ± 6	46 ± 7

[a] From Bona et al., 1978.

[b] PFC/10^7 mean of triplicate slides ± S.D.

[c] A48 is a BALB/c levan-binding IgA myeloma protein which does not carry E109 IdX.

[d] MOPC167 is a BALB/c phosphocholine IgA myeloma protein which does not carry E109 IdX.

response was heterogenous. After the second immunization when anti-Id autoantibodies were observed, some clonotypes were reduced in quantity or were absent. At this time, new clonotypes which had not been present after the first immunization were observed. Finally, after the third immunization, the IEF clonotype pattern of the first immunization and the new clonotypes which occurred after the appearance of anti-Id autoantibodies were detected together.

In summary, the results obtained in various antigenic systems, such as PC, bacterial levan, and *Micrococcus* polysaccharide, showed that Id-bearing antibodies which occur after immunization with conventional antigens are able to induce the production of anti-Id autoantibodies. This indicates that immunization with at least these three antigens activated two types of clones: one which produced IdX-bearing antibodies and another which produced anti-Id antibodies. The cyclic pattern of the kinetics of these two clones and the inverse fluctuation of their products clearly suggest the existence of a regulatory mechanism mediated by anti-Id antibodies. The antigen induces the production of IdX-bearing antibodies which in turn elicit the production of anti-Id antibodies. These later suppress the clones producing IdX-bearing antibodies. Therefore, these findings indicate that Id determinants, expressed on antibodies of a polyclonal immune response during which several clones were stimulated by the same antigen, persist a long time after antigenic stimulation. However, the same idiotypic determinants can be expressed on several clonotypes and on different Ig classes. In some antigenic systems new idiotypic specificities can be observed during the course of the immune response. The occurrence of these new idiotypic specificities during a secondary immune response can be related at least in part to the spontaneous appearance of anti-idiotypic autoantibodies produced in response to Ig secreted by the clones which have been activated in the early stages. In several experimental systems it has been shown that spontaneously occurring anti-Id autoantibodies suppress the Id⁺ component of the antibody response.

4

Expression of Idiotypes on B Cells

Bursa or bone marrow-derived (B) lymphocytes are responsible for the synthesis of antibodies. This function is genetically programmed and is generated independently of the presence of antigen. The progeny of one clone express a single V_H–V_L gene combination and, as a result, synthesize antibody specific for one particular antigen. B lymphocytes bear on their surface Ig receptors specific for antigen as well as a variety of non-immunoglobulin receptors, cytodifferentiation antigens, and the antigens encoded by the MHC. Thus B cells possess receptors for activated C3, Fc fragment, mitogens, hormones, chalones, and macrophage products. They express the histocompatibility and Ia antigens of the MHC locus and cytodifferentiation antigens which have been identified only on the B lineage (i.e. Lyb_3, Lyb_5, Lyb_7, MBLA, and PC antigens of murine B cells).

B lymphocytes appear to be heterogenous from a functional point of view. Thus, those B cells that give rise to antibody-producing cells can be divided into two subsets: a subset that requires cooperation with T-derived lymphocytes and another subset that is T-independent (TI). This latter is constituted by two distinct subsets: one which responds to TI-1 and another to TI-2 antigens. The heterogeneity of B cell populations with regard to their mitogenic responsiveness is also evident (Bona *et al.*, 1978). However, the common and most specific marker of B cells of all mammalian species is the Ig receptor which carries out the recognition function, the first specific event of any antibody response.

I. Expression of Idiotypes on Ig Receptor of B Cells

Ig receptor represents the specific marker of B lymphocyte populations. The Ig attached to the surface of lymphocytes present all the properties attributed to humoral antibodies.

They possess the ability to bind antigen and play an important role in the recognition process (Mäkelä, 1970), and they express the antigenic markers of various Ig classes (Coombs *et al.*, 1970a; Raff *et al.*, 1970) as well as the allotypic antigens carried by constant regions of Ig molecules (Pernis *et al.*, 1970; Coombs *et al.*, 1970b; Wernet *et al.*, 1972; Fu *et al.*, 1974c). McConnell *et al.* (1976) have shown that the murine B lymphocytes express the variable region (Fv) determinants of Ig molecules. They prepared a serum specific for framework determinants of the variable region by using as immunogen the Fv fragment of MOPC315 myeloma protein (IgA). An antisera against this Fv fragment was prepared in the rabbit. The presence of Fv determinants on the surface of lymphocytes was detected by incubation of lymphocytes with anti-Fv-purified antibodies and then staining with fluorescein-labeled goat anti-rabbit Ig. The antisera reacted with 44% lymph node cells and 2% of thymus-educated cells. This anti-Fv serum strongly inhibited the antigen-binding ability of sheep red blood cells (SRBC) to lymphocytes from mice immunized with sheep erythrocytes. By indirect immunofluorescence and rosette inhibition, Fv determinants were shown to be present on mouse lymphocytes. The percentage of peripheral lymphocytes which expressed Fv determinants (44%) was slightly greater than the usual range reported for Ig^+ cells in lymph node. By rosette inhibition study, it was shown that all SRBC-binding cells were inhibited by anti-Fv serum. This demonstrates that Fv determinants of humoral Ig are part of the antigen receptor of B cells. Claflin *et al.* (1974) have shown that antigen-binding receptors of B cells express idiotypic determinants. In normal mice (0.8 to 5) per 10^5 cells were able to bind phosphocholine (PC). The frequency of these PC-binding cells increases 100-fold after immunization with pneumococcal vaccine. This increase is paralleled by an increased anti-PC PFC response and of the titer of the PC antibodies. The Ig receptor of PC-binding cells was of the IgM class. Interestingly the PC-binding ability of these cells has been ablated by the anti-Id serum raised against PC-binding HOPC8 of myeloma protein. HOPC8, TEPC15 share T15IdX with anti-PC antibodies produced after immunization of BALB/c mice with R36A pneumococcal vaccine.

A more direct demonstration of the T15IdX on the receptor of lymphocytes was the enumeration of anti-idiotypic fluorescent cells. By this method Kohler *et al.* (1974) scored (30 to 45) per 10^4 spleen cells stained with anti-Id antibodies. The number of cells which express T15IdX is one order of magnitude more than the number of PC antigen-binding cells. Kohler *et al.* (1974) explained this discrepancy with the argument that the T15I idiotype is not necessarily related only to PC-binding cells, but could also be expressed on other cells which do not bind PC.

Binz and Wigzell (1975a) have shown that B cells reactive to alloantigens express the Id determinants of antialloantigen antibodies. Similarly, we have shown that rabbit Ig^+ cells which have been selected by the mixed agglutination technique and which are stimulated by NWSM were stained by peroxidase-labeled F(ab')2 fragments of anti-RNase Id antibodies. In these experiments, the same rabbit immunized with RNase was the donor of cells and of antibodies used to prepare anti-Id antibodies. In addition, the cells which have been stained with anti-Id antibodies were stained with a goat antiserum specific for framework determinants of rabbit-Ig molecules (Cazenave *et al.*, 1977a). Therefore, it appears that Ig receptors of B cells express all the antigenic determinants attributed to circulating antibodies. Both idiotypic and framework antigenic determinants of V region of Ig molecules have been identified on B cells. The association of idiotypes with the membrane of murine plasmocytoma and lymphocytes of human Waldenstrom macroglobulinemia, multiple myeloma, and leukemic cells is well documented. These tumor B cells originated from a single cell which proliferates and generates malignant cell clones.

Sugai *et al.* (1974) have prepared anti-Id antibodies against a monoclonal IgM of B/W mice with 141 lymphoma. These antibodies were specific for the Fv antigenic determinants of monoclonal IgM. The presence of Id determinants on Ig of lymphoma cells was studied by staining with fluoresceinated reagents and by cytotoxic assay. More than 90% of lymphoma cells in the progressive phase of the disease expressed Id determinants on their membrane.

Haughton *et al.* (1978) prepared anti-Id antibodies against the myeloma lysates of CH1 tumor cells which do not secrete protein. The presence of Id determinants on the surface IgM (sIgM) of these CH1 tumor cells was studied by fluorescence and cytotoxic assays. About

90% of cells were positive for both IgM and idiotype as was established by both methods.

These results indicate that sIg of myeloma or lymphoma cells express Id determinants of monoclonal proteins secreted by these cells.

Similar conclusions were drawn subsequent to the studies on the expression of Id determinants on the lymphocytes of human B tumors, such as Waldenstrom macroglobulinemia, multiple myeloma, and chronic lymphoid leukemia. Wernet *et al.* (1972) using a cytotoxic assay have demonstrated the presence of Id determinants on a high number of lymphocytes from patients with Waldenstrom macroglobulinemia. Anti-Id serum and complement (C) killed 42% of cells from the patient with macroglobulinemia, whereas it was not cytotoxic on the lymphocytes from health donors (0.4%). The anti-human-μ serum and C killed 44% of cells from the patient and 9.7% of cells from normal donor. It seems likely, according to these results, that the majority of sIg lymphocytes of the patient with macroglobulinemia have sIgM of the same idiotype as that of his serum macroglobulins used to raise the anti-Id serum.

Multiple myeloma is another B cell malignancy which involves the B cell and plasma cells from bone marrow. There are several reports which showed that plasma cells from patients with multiple myeloma present a high percentage of sIg$^+$ cells and that these sIg react with antisera to Id determinants of myeloma proteins (Lindstrom *et al.,* 1973; Mellstadt *et al.,* 1974; Abdou and Abdou, 1975; Preud'homme *et al.,* 1977). Holm *et al.* (1977) have shown that varying numbers of blood lymphocytes from untreated IgG myeloma patients have been stained with F(ab')2 fragment of rabbit anti-Id and anti-human IgG antibodies. The sIg Id$^+$ cells generally disappeared during the remission phase of the disease, after treatment. These Id$^+$ sIg are not passively absorbed on the surface of lymphocytes since they regenerated in culture after the trypsin treatment (Mellstadt *et al.,* 1974) and they were not found on normal cells incubated with high amounts of myeloma proteins (Holm *et al.,* 1977). Id determinants of myeloma subjects were identified on three categories of lymphocytes: atypical small lymphocytes, atypical lymphoblasts, and atypical plasma cells.

There is a close relationship between Id determinants expressed on sIg and the Ig class of myeloma protein. In a patient with IgD myeloma protein, about 70% of circulating B lymphocytes expressed

IgD. Anti-Id serum raised against IgD myeloma protein cocapped Id^+ IgD receptor (Kubagawa et al., 1980). In the light of these results it appears that sIg of lymphocytes and plasma cells in multiple myeloma share Id determinants of myeloma protein secreted by these cells. Certain cases of chronic lymphocytic leukemia (CLL) are also associated with the occurrence of monoclonal Ig, as in multiple myeloma. Fu et al. (1974) have shown that the majority of lymphocytes from CLL subjects possess sIgM and sIgD. Fu et al. (1974) prepared an anti-Id serum against a serum monoclonal band from a patient with CLL. In this case, the fluoresceinated Fab fragment of anti-Id antibodies stained 68–73% of the cells. The same number of cells (67–74%) were stained with anti-IgM and (56–69%) with anti-IgD. The staining of cells with anti-Id serum was specific since it was inhibited with serum from the patient but not with normal serum. Both sIgM and sIgD expressed Id determinants since they were cocapped with anti-Id serum (Fu et al., 1974c).

The presence of Id determinants of serum monoclonal IgM bands has been identified on a lymphoid blast cell line derived from two patients with CLL (Hurley et al., 1978). In this study several lines were obtained from peripheral blood lymphocytes and spleen. Only a few of these lines were stained with anti-Id antibodies, indicating that other lines derived from nonleukemic B clones. The anti-Id sera stained sIg of small lymphocytes and few plasma cells. The Id^+ sIg lymphoid lines secrete in the culture IgM which expressed Id determinants of monoclonal bands as was demonstrated by both HA and hemagglutination inhibition (HI) assays. One of the Id^+ sIg leukemic lymphoid lines was cloned in soft agar. All the clones which have been obtained secreted IgM which shared the Id determinants of the monoclonal IgM band. Similarly, a great proportion of the progeny of these clones were stained with anti-Id, anti-IgM, and anti-IgD antibodies.

These data, taken collectively, show that Id determinants of monoclonal Ig secreted by murine plasmocytoma as well as various human malignant B cells are expressed on the sIg of lymphocytes.

The presence of Id determinants on the surface of tumor B cells is very important since they can serve as sites for anti-Id antibodies. In fact, myeloma cells are not simply autonomous malignant cells, but instead can respond to immunoregulatory signals as will be illustrated in the sections below.

II. Dependence of Expression of Idiotypes on Site of Localization of Lymphocytes within Lymphoid Tissue and B Lymphocyte Subsets

There are few reports on the variation of B cell repertoire in peripheral lymphoid organs and various subsets of B lymphocytes. Gerhardt and Cebra (1979) have studied the frequency of the precursors of anti-PC and the expression of T15IdX in the spleen and Peyer's patches. A majority of BALB/c splenic B cells specific for PC belong to T15 clonotype. In fact, anti-T15 idiotypic antibodies inhibit more than 90% of anti-PC PFC of BALB/c mice immunized with a 36A *Pneumococcus*. By contrast, most anti-PC antibody-forming cells of Peyer's patches secrete antibodies which do not bear T15IdX. This significant difference in the T15$^+$ fraction of anti-PC response between spleen and Peyer's patches probably can be related to the antigenic environment of the gut. Interestingly, mice infested orally with *Ascaris sum* (which bear PC antigenic determinants) produce anti-PC antibodies, but the T15$^+$ component of this response is very small (19%). Furthermore, while in the spleen the majority of the T15$^+$ and anti-PC antibodies belong to IgM class, in the Peyer's patches 30–50% of anti-PC antibodies belong to IgA class. The α dominance of the Peyer's patch B cell response represents a general phenomenon, since immunization with inulin or DNP generates more clones secreting only IgA. However, the α-isotype dominance of the Peyer's patch lymphocyte response is not strictly related to only the gut antigenic microenvironment. Gut B lymphocytes retain the ability preferentially to produce IgA even after transfer to an irradiated recipient. Gerhart and Cebra (1979) infused sublethally irradiated C.B20 mice (H-2^d, IgC-h^b) with BALB/c (H-2^d, IgC-h^a) Peyer's patch lymphocytes and then determined the frequency of α isotype anti-PC precursors in the spleen of the recipient mice. They found that BALB/c cells retained their ability to make predominantly IgA-anti-PC PFC. Thus, the potential of gut B cells to make IgA is not transient, but is genetically programmed. It, therefore, appears that variation of *C-h* gene expression of B cells is closely related to the organ origin of B cells. The dominance of α isotype on B cells in Peyer's patches can be related to the abundance of α-isotype-specific helper T cells. The helper T cells seem to be required in the switching of cIgM$^+$mIgD$^+$ cells to IgA-producing cells. However, dominance of the α isotype response in the gut suggests a particular and preferential translocation of V genes to the C-α gene than to other C-h genes.

It seems that the IgM anti-PC response is particular for a subset of B lymphocytes which is under the control of sex-linked genes. Mond *et al.* (1977) have studied the expression of T15IdX and anti-PC response in male F_1 hybrids (CBA/N × BALB/c and CBA/N × DBA/2N) which bear the X-linked defect of CBA/N mice (xid). This defect results in the failure of the development of a subpopulation of B lymphocytes which is found in normal mice. The mutant strain CBA/N or the male F_1 hybrids do not respond to T-independent TI_2 antigens as TNP-Ficoll, TNP-dextran, TNP-levan. Male F_1 hybrids from mating of CBA/N × DNA/2N or CBA/N × BALB/c failed to develop T15 titers after immunization with T-dependent antigens (e.g., PC-DNA) or T-independent antigens (e.g., PC-*Brucella abortus* or R36A pneumococcal vaccine). After immunization with PC-OVA, the female F_1 hybrids have more than 8×10^5 anti-PC PFC/spleen, while the males have none. It appears that the mice with xid defect are unable to develop an IgM or IgG $T15^+$ anti-PC response. However, recently Kishimato *et al.* (1979) have shown that the mice bearing xid-defect gene can develop an IgE anti-PC response, indicating that the structural V genes which control the expression of T15IdX and the PC specificity are present in these mice and can be expressed in other B cell subsets or lineages.

These data indicate that V genes which control the specificity of the B cell repertoire are expressed on lymphocytes lodged in various lymphoid organs or which belong to various B subsets. However, there are important differences in the expression of the V genes, which can be dependent on the lodging of lymphocytes in various lymphoid organs as well as on the development of various subsets of B lymphocytes.

III. Activation of Precursors of Antibody-Forming Cells by Anti-idiotypic Antibodies

The Ig receptor of B cells expresses Id determinants of antibody molecules secreted by these cells. These Id determinants might serve as sites for anti-Id antibodies. Several findings have been reported which show that interaction of anti-Id antibodies with B cells led to their activation and differentiation into antibody-secreting cells in the absence of antigen. This interaction mimics the binding of antigen to Ig receptor. Trenkner and Riblet (1975) have studied the effects of S107Id antibodies on the anti-PC response. S107, like TEPC15 or HOPC8, is an IgA_k PC-binding myeloma protein which shares the same IdX. The effects of rabbit and A/HeJ anti-S107IdX antibodies were studied *in vitro*. After incubation of BALB/c and BAB.14 spleen cells with various amounts of anti-Id antibodies, the anti-PC PFC response was compared to that induced by R36A vaccine. Rabbit anti-S107 antibodies caused an anti-PC PFC response, whereas A/HeJ anti-Id antibodies failed to stimulate the precursor of anti-PC antibody-secreting cells. This stimulation was specific, since the spleen cells of C.AL9 mice were not stimulated. C.AL9 mice are BALB/c H-2^d congenic mice which have Igh-V^e and IgC-h^e and do not express S107IdX encoded by *IgV-h^a* genes. The magnitude of the anti-PC response elicited by rabbit anti-Id antibodies in the culture of BALB/c and BAB.14 spleen cells was about half of that induced by stimulation of cultures with R36A vaccine.

The inability to obtain induction of the anti-PC PFC response with mouse (A/HeJ) anti-S107Id antibodies was interpreted by Trenker and Riblet (1975) as a lack of strong carrier determinants recognized by helper T cells on A/HeJ antibodies. However, an alternative explanation can be provided by the discovery of Claflin and Davie (1975b) that, while rabbit anti-T15Id antibodies interact with combining-site Id determinants, A/HeJ anti-T15Id antibodies interact with framework-associated Id determinants. It, therefore, appears that perhaps only anti-Id antibodies against combining site-associated Id determinants can mimic the antigen.

The F(ab')$_2$ fragments of rabbit anti-S107IdX antibodies as well as A/He anti-Id antibodies failed to activate the precursor of anti-PC cells. This finding suggested that the Fc fragment is required for the activation of B cells. The Fc fragment can be required either to ensure the participation of T cells or to be bound to both Ig and Fc receptors of B cells. In the latter case, it would mimic the "repetitive antigenic determinants" of T-independent antigens, i.e., the conformation of PC antigenic determinants on the cell wall of R36A *Pneumococcus*.

Indeed, in additional experiments the authors have shown that the second signal provided by an Fc receptor can be replaced by T cells or lipopolysaccharide (LPS). These results suggest that anti-Id antibodies behave as T-independent antigens and can trigger anti-PC cells, whereas F(ab')2 fragments of these antibodies require a second activator signal. Interestingly, Kohler *et al.* (1978) have observed a requirement for Fc fragments of mouse anti-Id antibodies in the induction of idiotype suppression in the PC system, indicating that the binding of the anti-Id antibody molecule to both Ig and Fc receptor can cause either activation or tolerance. Eichmann and Rajewsky (1975) have shown that anti-Id antibodies, as well as antigen, can prime B cells, and only that B compartment which expresses the idiotype can be activated. They found that the IgG_1 fraction of anti-A5AId antibodies can presensitize the A/J mice for a secondary response challenged by *Streptococcus* A.

These results suggest again that anti-Id antibodies mimic the binding of antigen to Ig receptor. It should be mentioned that in both antigenic systems (i.e., PC and *Streptococcus* A) the anti-Id antibodies which were able to mimic antigen were heterologous antibodies and were specific for the combining-site-associated Id determinants. In bacterial levan system we have not been able to stimulate the production of $E109IdX^+$ anti-inulin or anti-levan antibodies after the administration *in vivo* or after *in vitro* culture of BALB/c spleen cells with A/He anti-E109IdX antibodies. However, when the spleen cells from BALB/c mice presensitized *in vivo* with anti-Id antibodies were cultured *in vitro* with NWSM we detected in the medium fluid $E109^+$ anti-levan and anti-inulin antibodies (Bona, 1979b) (Fig. 4.1). In this system it appeared that only the presence of a mitogenic signal can trigger the precursors primed *in vivo* by anti-Id antibodies.

IV. T-Independent Idiotype Suppression

Suppression of synthesis of immunoglobulins has been achieved by antisera directed against antigenic determinants of Ig molecules. This suppression of synthesis of Ig was obtained both *in vitro* after incubation of lymphocytes with anti-Ig antisera or subsequent to parenteral administration of these antisera.

In vivo administration of anti-μ antibodies invariably results in severe suppression of B cell functions, reduction or elimination of plasma cells, absence of germinal centers, and inhibition of synthesis of Ig. The inhibition of Ig classes is accompanied by a nonspecific inhibition of synthesis of the antibody responses for various antigens as a result of suppression of IgM-bearing precursors (see review by Stanislawski, 1981). Similarly, *in vitro* incubation of lymphocytes with

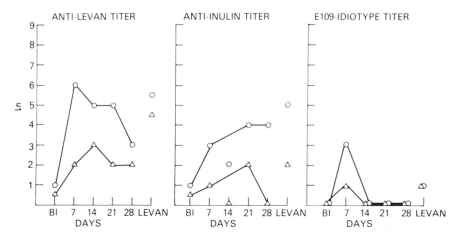

Fig. 4.1. *In vitro* stimulation of production of anti-levan, anti-inulin antibodies carrying E109 idiotype by spleen cells of BALB/c mice. BI = Nonimmunized mice; log 2 = titer (ln); ○, cells originating from BALB/c mice immunized with 10 μg bacterial levan; △, cells originating from BALB/c mice treated with 0.1 ml A/He anti-E109 anti-idiotype serum. 5×10^7 cells were cultured in RPMI 1640 medium supplemented with 10% fetal calf serum (FCS) (10^7/ml), and the supernatant harvested after 78 hours was concentrated 20×. Anti-levan and anti-inulin titers were determined by agglutination of levan- and inulin-coated sheep erythrocytes (SRBC) and E109-idiotype titer by inhibition of hemagglutination of A/He anti-E109 serum and U61-coated SRBC.

anti-IgM leads to the inhibition of synthesis of Ig in the culture despite B lymphocyte proliferation and incorporation of [³H]thymidine (see review by Bona, 1981).

Injection of anti-allotype antibodies during the neonatal period or following transplacental transmission from mothers immunized against paternal allotypes causes a long-lasting suppression of the corresponding allotype (see review by Horng *et al.*, 1981). Similarly, *in vitro* incubation of lymphocytes with anti-allotype antibodies causes a specific suppression of synthesis of Ig carrying the corresponding allotype in spite of the ability of these lymphocytes to incorporate [³H]thymidine and to differentiate into lymphoblasts (see review by Bona and Cazenave, 1981).

Both *in vivo* and *in vitro* induced idiotypic suppression is highly specific. Indeed, only the clones which bear the corresponding idiotype are suppressed. This contrasts with isotypic and allotype suppression, which are nonspecific, since the ability of Ig synthesis of various clones which secrete Ig-bearing isotypic and allotypic antigenic determinants is inhibited.

The study of idiotype suppression in adult animals induced by parenteral administration of anti-Id antibodies suggests that suppression can be achieved by two different mechanisms. A T-mediated idiotype suppression occurs in which the anti-Id antibodies generate suppressor T cells which can exert their effect on helper T cells or directly on B cells and inhibit the Id^+ component of the antibody response. In this case, the anti-Id antibodies behave as would an antigen, inducing the occurrence of antigen suppressor T cells. The second category is represented by direct idiotype suppression of the precursor of antibody-forming cells as a result of interaction between anti-Id antibodies and Id^+-bearing antigen receptors of the B cell. In this case, the anti-Id antibodies behave as T-independent tolerogenic signals which cause the unresponsiveness of B cells. This kind of idiotype suppression is T-independent and is not cell-mediated.

A. Direct Idiotype Suppression Induced by Homologous Anti-Id Antibodies

The main data concerning this type of suppression come from studies performed in mice and rabbits. In the PC antigenic systems, idiotype suppression was obtained by the following.

1. *In vitro* pretreatment of BALB/c spleen cells with A/He anti-T15IdX antibodies (Kohler, 1975).

2. *In vivo* administration of anti-T15IdX antibodies in BALB/c mice, followed by challenge with R36A pneumococcal vaccine (Cosenza and Kohler, 1971).

3. Immunization of BALB/c mice with HOPC8 myeloma protein, followed by challenge with PC antigens (Rowley *et al.,* 1978), since T15IdX response is dominant the inhibition of total anti-PC response was over 90%. This inhibition is specific since anti-MOPC167Id antibodies had no inhibitory activity. MOPC167, like TEPC15 or HOPC8, is IgA_k, PC-binding myeloma protein which bears an IdI which is not expressed on BALB/c anti-PC antibodies (Cosenza and Kohler, 1972).

4. The anti-TNP and anti-SRBC response was identical in normal BALB/c mice or pretreated with A/He anti-T15IdX antibodies (Cosenza and Kohler, 1972; Rowley *et al.,* 1978).

By contrast to the long-term suppression induced in neonatal mice, the suppression in adults is of brief duration. By 4–5 weeks after completion of treatment and immunization, half the mice have recovered from suppression, and by 6 weeks all the mice responded normally to R36A pneumococcal vaccine. The adult idiotype suppression of the T15IdX$^+$ anti-PC antibody response is not compensated by an increase of T15$^-$ anti-PC antibodies as was observed following neonatal suppression.

The effects of *in vivo* complementary antibody responses (i.e., anti-IdX and anti-PC) were explored by Rowley *et al.* (1978) in BALB/c mice immunized simultaneously with PC-KLH and HOPC8. Both responses were measured by enumerating the PFC specific for PC and HOPC8IdX and by assaying serum antibody levels to PC and HOPC8. As expected, the sera from mice immunized to have low titers of anti-PC hemagglutinins and high titers of anti-HOPC8Id antibodies inhibited the anti-PC PFC. These mice exhibited a low number of anti-PC cells. By contrast the sera from mice immunized to have high response for both PC and HOPCIdX failed to inhibit the anti-PC PFC response and themselves exhibited both normal anti-PC and HOPC8 PFC response. The absence of reciprocal regulation observed in this later experiment can be due to the formation of complexes which are cleared before exerting their effect on antibody-forming cells. The possible occurrence of anti- (anti-Id) antibodies was not investigated, and therefore no available data exist on the possible second degree of Id–anti-Id reaction which could appear and disturb the regulatory ability of various components of the network. The unresponsiveness of the adult mice following pretreatment with anti-T15Id antibodies results from a reversible blockade of the receptors of precursors of anti-PC cells. The spleen cells from adult suppressed mice cultured *in vitro* with R34A vaccine responded like cells from normal animals (Kohler *et al.* 1974). This observation indicated that during culture period the cells cleared from their surface with anti-Id receptor complex and the newly regenerated receptor was able to bind PC, and then this binding triggered the precursor of the anti-PC antibody-forming cells. This explanation was also supported by staining experiments in which fluoresceinated anti-T15IdX antibodies were used. These antibodies stained 25 to 35 per 10^4 cells in normal mice, and no cells were stained in suppressed mice. If the cells from suppressed mice were cultured for 15 minutes again only 1 per 10^4 cells were stained. However, after 4 hours of incubation the number of stained cells in suppressed animals was equal to the number of cells stained in normal mice (Kohler, 1975). These results suggest that the interaction between anti-Id antibodies with membrane Ig receptor of anti-PC cells turns off the synthesis of anti-PC antibodies. It seems that anti-Id antibodies exert a direct effect on the precursors in this system. The most important findings which support the direct suppressive mechanism of anti-T15Id antibodies were provided by the experiments of Strayer *et al.* (1975). They showed that after infusion of a mixture of cells from normal and suppressed animals into lethally irradiated BALB/c mice which were then immunized with R36A pneumococcal vaccine, the anti-PC response of reconstituted recipients was identical to that of irradiated mice infused with only normal cells. So far no evidence exists to suggest that A/He anti-T15 antibodies generate after the administration *in vivo* suppressor T cells which mediate the Id suppression in adult. However, DuClos and Kim (1977) showed that cells sensitive to anti-Thy 1.2 + C treatment, originating from 6- to 8-week-old neonatally suppressed mice, can inhibit the *in vitro* induced PFC response of normal spleen cells. Kim (1979) was able to induce suppressor cells *in vitro* by incubating the spleen cells from normal animals with anti-T15Id antibodies and R36A pneumococcal vaccine.

These new findings suggest to the investigators the existence of precursors of suppressor T cells which can be activated by anti-T15IdX antibodies and/or antigen. Why such cells cannot be activated *in vivo* after administration of anti-Id antibodies and R36A vaccine is unclear. Homologous anti-T15IdX antibodies belonging to various classes of Ig were efficient in the induction of *in vivo* adult suppression. However, Kohler *et al.* (1979) have found that F(ab')2-fragment preparations of mouse anti-Id antibodies did not suppress the anti-PC response. This suggests that a cross-linking of surface Fc and Ig receptors is required for the induction of idiotype suppression. It is not clear by which mechanism the cross-linking of Ig and Fc receptor by an anti-Id antibody molecule delivers a tolerogenic signal. In fact, the dependent stimulation of Fc receptor by binding of Ig molecules or of Ig receptor following interaction with anti-Ig antibodies stimulates the differentiation of small B lymphocytes into blasts and increases their [^{3}H]thymidine incorporation (Weigle and Berman, 1979; Sieckmann *et al.,* 1978; Sidman and Unanue, 1978).

The suppression of IdXs of anti-inulin and anti-levan antibodies provided another clear example of T-independent idiotype suppression (Bona *et al.*, 1979a). The response of BALB/c mice to bacterial levan (BL) was markedly influenced by pretreatment with anti-E109 antibodies, which contain anti-IdXG and anti-IdXA antibody. Thus, pretreatment of BALB/c or other allotype Igl[a] congenic strains of mice with anti-E109IdX antibodies leads to a profound suppression of the production of anti-inulin antibody response to immunization with BL when assessed by hemagglutination (Fig. 4.2), enumeration of plaque-forming cells, and isoelectric focusing (Fig. 4.3). These mice make little anti-inulin antibody until 60 days after immunization and, similarly, fail to express IdX-bearing molecules among the anti-BL antibodies that they do produce. Suppression caused by pretreatment with anti-E109 is specific, since no alteration in the anti-TNP antibody response was observed in BALB/c mice pretreated with anti-E109 and then immunized with TNP-Ficoll alone or together with bacterial levan (Table 4.1).

The finding that suppression extends to both the ability to transfer

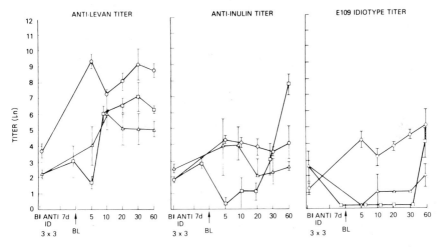

Fig. 4.2. Kinetics of serum anti-BL and anti-inulin (Inu) responses and serum IdX titers after immunization of normal or idiotype suppressed BALB/c mice with BL. The left and center panels show the kinetics of the hemagglutinin titer against BL-SRBC and Inu-SRBC, respectively. The right panel shows the kinetics of the levels of the E109IdX in the sera of the same mice. O—O, immunization with 10 μg BL; △—△, pretreatment with anti-E109 not followed by immunization with BL; □—□, pretreatment with anti-E109 followed 7 days later by immunization with BL. Each point represents the mean ± SE of the determinations performed on five mice. From Bona *et al.*, 1979c.

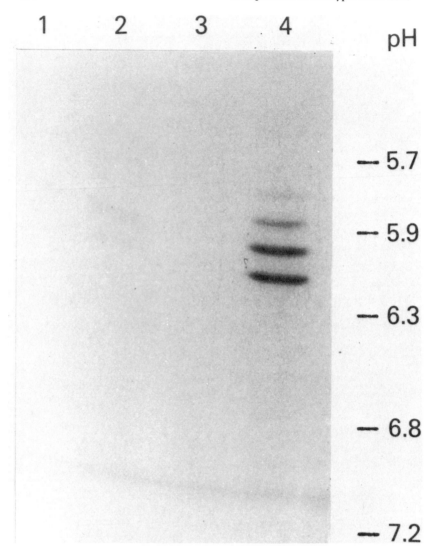

Fig. 4.3. Isoelectric focusing pattern of sera of adult normal and suppressed BALB/c mice immunized with BL. Twenty microliters of pooled serum from five individual mice was applied to each lane. The radioactive overlay consisted of inulin-[^{125}I]BSA and the film was exposed for 3 days. The bands of pH 7.1 and 7.7 probably represent binding of label by non-anti-inulin antibodies. (1) Normal adult BALB/c mice 5 days after immunization with 10 μg BL. (2) Adult BALB/c mice injected three times at 3-day intervals, with 0.1 ml A/He anti-E109 idiotype antiserum and immunized 7 days after the completion of pretreatment with 10 μg BL. From Bona *et al.*, 1979b.

TABLE 4.1

Responses to **BL** and TNP-Ficoll of Normal and E109IdX-Suppressed **BALB/c Mice**[a]

Immunization of mice			PFC Response		
			Anti-BL		Anti-TNP
Anti-E109 treatment[b]	Bacterial levan (BL) (10 µg)	TNP-Ficoll (20 µg)	PFC/10^7 cells	% E109 positive	(PFC/10^7 cells)
−[c]	+	−	890 ± 134	46 ± 8	273 ± 82
+[d]	+	−	281 ± 71	13 ± 7	432 ± 86
−	+	+	2569 ± 361	39 ± 8	4194 ± 339
+	+	+	432 ± 147	13 ± 10	7359 ± 2150
−	−	+	183 ± 107	40 ± 12	3554 ± 297
+	−	+	199 ± 63	25 ± 8	5774 ± 346

[a] From Bona et al., 1979c.
[b] Adult BALB/c mice were injected three times at 3-day intervals with 0.1 ml anti-E109 anti-idiotypic serum and immunized 7 days later with BL, TNP-Ficoll, or both. The response in these mice as well as in normal mice was tested 5 days after immunization.
[c] No treatment with antiserum.
[d] Treatment with antiserum.

responses and to develop PFC is strong evidence in favor of a true suppression at the cellular level rather than a simple clearance of IdX[+] anti-inulin antibody by anti-idiotypic antibodies. The suppression of E109IdX-bearing cells appears to be largely independent of thymic influence since it occurs in *nu/nu* BALB/c mice (Fig. 4.4). The experiments in which we attempted to transfer idiotypic suppression by cells have clearly shown that the mechanism of this kind of suppression results from the binding of anti-E109 antibody to precursors bearing membrane Ig which possesses the IdX. In these experiments BALB/c mice irradiated with 650 rads have been reconstituted with spleen cells from normal BALB/c or BALB/c mice pretreated with anti-Id antibodies or with a 1 : 1 mixture of normal or pretreated cells. When normal BALB/c spleen cells have been infused 41% of anti-levan and 90% of anti-inulin PFC expressed E109IdX. A markedly lower E109[+] component of both responses was observed when the cells from suppressed mice have been transferred alone. Transfer of a 1 : 1 mixture of cells from normal and suppressed animals did not result in suppression of the ability to make E109[+] anti-levan and anti-inulin antibodies (Table 4.2). The results of these transfer experiments indicate that the suppression of precursors of E109-secreting cells is T

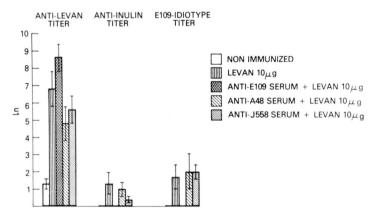

Fig. 4.4. The humoral response to 10 μg of BL of *nu/nu* BALB/c mice pretreated with various anti-idiotype sera. BL-SRBC titer (left panel), Inu-SRBC titer (center panel), and the level of the serum E109IdX (right panel). Each column represents the mean ± S.E. of determinations performed on five mice. Note that anti-inulin titers and E109-idiotype titers of "nonimmunized" and of "anti-E109 serum + levan 10 μg" groups are zero. From Bona *et al.*, 1979c.

TABLE 4.2

Inability to Transfer E109IdX Suppression[a]

BALB/c mice irradiated with 650 rads and infused with	Anti-BL PFC/10⁷		Anti-Inu PFC/10⁷		Titer (ln)		
	Total	% E109+	Total	% E109+	Anti-BL (HA)	Anti-Inu (HA)	E109IdX (HI)
No cells	13 ± 2	15 ± 13	12 ± 1	75 ± 10	1.5 ± 0.5	1.0 ± 0	0.5 ± 0.5
10⁸ normal spleen cells (a)	1480 ± 109	41 ± 15	683 ± 31	90 ± 12	6.3 ± 1.3	3.0 ± 0	4.0 ± 0.5
5 × 10⁷ spleen cells from BALB/c mice pretreated thrice with anti-E109 antibodies (b)	880 ± 125	0	73 ± 18	10 ± 5	4.3 ± 0.3	0.6 ± 0.8	1.0 ± 1.0
5 × 10⁷ (a) + 5 × 10⁷ (b)	1046 ± 125	20 ± 6	290 ± 23	79 ± 6	5.0 ± 1.0	1.5 ± 0.5	2.0 ± 0
5 × 10⁷ (a) + 5 × 10⁷ (b) [(b) pretreated with anti-Thy-1.2 + C]	1006 ± 46	22 ± 12	296 ± 9	84 ± 5	4.0 ± 2.0	2.0 ± 1.0	3.0 ± 0

[a] Each group consisted of five mice which were immunized with 10 μg BL 1 day after transfer of cells.

independent and directly results from the binding of antibodies to Ig receptor bearing IdX of the precursors.

We have also studied the expression of IdX and IdI of XRPC24 (X24) galactan-binding myeloma protein in BALB/c mice pretreated with A/He anti-X24Id antibodies. Adult BALB/c mice have been pretreated at 3-day intervals with anti-Id antisera and then immunized with gum ghatti. In the spleen of these mice we enumerated the anti-galactan PFC, and in the sera we measured the level of X24IdI and IdX. No differences were observed between the anti-galactan response of normal and suppressed mice (Table 4.3). We have no adequate explanation for the failure to induce idiotype suppression in adult BALB/c mice, since with the same A/He anti-X24 serum we obtained a strong suppression of anti-galactan as well as X24IdI and -IdX when these antibodies have been injected in the neonatal period.

TABLE 4.3

Kinetics of Serum X24IdX after Immunization with Gum Ghatti of Normal or Idiotype Suppressed BALB/c Mice[a]

No. of mice	Day 0	Day 7	Day 21	Day 60	Day 90
Level of X24IdX in normal BALB/c mice					
1	0.029	0.0012	0.03	0.03	0.0115
2	0.42	0.005	0.051	0.02	0.021
3	0.011	0.0011	0.022	0.012	0.005
4	0.16	0.01	0.033	0.018	0.0069
5	0.16	0.006	0.03	0.021	0.003
6	0.047	0.011	0.033	0.00	0.016
7	0.082	0.05	0.041	0.025	0.0094
8	0.2	0.009	0.004	0.018	0.0076
9	0.27	0.03	0.038	ND[b]	0.0088
Level of X24IdX in BALB/c mice pretreated with A/He antiX24IdX antiserum					
1	0.12	0.07	0.02	0.87	0.019
2	0.07	0.026	0.038	0.46	0.008
3	0.08	0.027	0.082	0.03	0.023
4	0.14	0.027	0.036	0.02	0.049
5	0.16	0.0522	0.016	0.034	0.012
6	0.03	0.0022	0.022	0.003	0.0119
7	0.064	0.016	0.038	0.02	0.015
8	0.026	0.022	0.029	0.034	0.038
9	0.03	0.027	0.009	0.004	0.013

[a] Values = serum dilution giving 50% control binding.
[b] ND, not done.

Bordenave (1975) obtained idiotype suppression of a secondary response in rabbits, using homologous anti-Id serum. He prepared anti-Id antibodies against anti-*S. abortus equi* antibodies obtained after a primary immunization. Three weeks before a booster injection of bacteria, the rabbits received injections of anti-Id antibodies prepared from their own serum harvested after the priming. The administration of these anti-Id antibodies led to the suppression of some idiotypes. However, a few idiotypes already present in the preimmune serum have not been suppressed. A new set of anti-Id antibodies has been prepared against the "nonsuppressed idiotypes," and this serum was used for a "second" suppression. After these two successive suppressions, no new idiotypes were observed. According to Bordenave (1975), anti-idiotype antibodies probably suppressed the idiotype production by combining with the Ig receptor of memory cells bearing the corresponding Id determinants and thus the cells have been diverted from idiotype production.

The results presented herein indicate that the suppression of precursors of IdX-secreting cells in PC and levan–inulin system in mice and *S. abortus equi* in rabbits is T independent and directly results from the interaction between anti-Id antibodies and the Ig receptor of the precursors. This interaction mimics the binding of T-independent antigen to a B cell Ig receptor and in the absence of T cells leads to the induction of tolerance. Mouse or rabbit Ig are weak immunogens, and thus the T cell help mounted by recognition of allotypic determinants is very low; thus the interaction between anti-Id and receptor leads to tolerance rather than to stimulation. However, since it is known that only high doses of T-independent antigens cause tolerance, it seems likely that the amount of anti-Id antibodies persist a long time to permit a blockage of the receptors of the precursors. The cross-linking of Fc and Ig receptors by anti-Id antibodies or anti-Id, -IdX-bearing antibody complexes could represent an alternative explanation for the ability of anti-Id antibody to deliver a tolerogenic signal. In fact, Kohler *et al.* (1979) have shown that $F(ab')_2$ fragments of anti-Id antibodies failed to cause idiotype suppression.

B. Indirect Idiotypic Suppression

During the study of idiotype suppression in the levan–inulin system we observed inhibition by anti-E109IdX antibodies of an E109⁻ antibody response. We called this new phenomenon "indirect suppression." BALB/c mice immunized with BL produce two families of antibodies. One binds only $\beta(2\rightarrow6)$fructosan and does not express the IdXs of the inulin-binding myeloma protein. A second family of antibodies binds $\beta(2\rightarrow6)$- and $\beta(2\rightarrow1)$fructosan and expresses IdXs. The pretreatment with anti-E109 serum resulted in a drastic decrease in the anti-BL titer; while the normal mice had a titer of 9.5 ln units (1 : 724) the suppressed mice had only 2.1 (1 : 4.3). Thus, 168-fold difference in titer is greater than would be expected from the fact that no more than 50% of anti-BL antibodies express E109IdX. In addition we have observed that *in vitro,* anti-E109IdX antibody pretreatment leads to a decrease of the anti-TNP antibody response elicited by TNP-BL. In these experiments 10^7 BALB/c spleen cells were incubated for 24 hours with nothing, normal A/He Ig, or A/He anti-E109Ig and then stimulated with BL, NWSM, or TNP coupled with *B. abortus* (TNA-BA). After 3 days' culture, the polyclonal effect of BL and NWSM and the specific stimulation with TNP-BA was assessed by enumerating the anti-TNP and anti-inulin PFC. It was observed that the $E109^+$ component of the anti-inulin PFC response was strongly inhibited by preincubation with anti-E109IdX antibodies. This was true for stimulation with BL, which probably represents a specific stimulation, as well as after stimulation with NWSM and TNP-BL (presumably representing polyclonal activation). More interestingly, the polyclonal effect of BL with respect to stimulation of anti-TNP PFC was strongly inhibited, whereas the ability of NWSM or TNP-BA to stimulate anti-TNP PFC responses was not affected by the preincubation of cells with anti-E109 (Table 4.4). In further experiments, the effects of anti-E109IdX antibodies have been studied on the anti-TNP response induced by TNP-BL and TNP-inulin in order to investigate the effects of blockade of the E109IdX-bearing receptor of the precurosr of anti-E109IdX antibodies.

Preincubation of BALB/c spleen cells with anti-E109IdX antibodies inhibited the response to TNP-levan or TNP-inulin but had no effect on TNP-LPS. In control experiments we have studied the effect of anti-A48Id and anti-MOPC384Id antibodies. ABPC48 (A48) is a myeloma protein which binds only $\beta(2\rightarrow6)$fructosan and carries an unrelated IdI. MOPC384 is specific for α-methyl-β-D-galactoside (the immunodominant sugar of LPS of *S. tranoroa*) and bears an unrelated IdX. The preincubation of cells with anti-A48Id antibodies inhibits only the anti-TNP response induced by TNP-BL and did not affect the response induced by TNP-inulin or TNP-LPS. Anti-384Id an-

TABLE 4.4

Effect of Anti-E109 Idiotype Antibodies on Specific and Polyclonal Responses to BL[a]

Additions to culture		Response (PFC/culture) anti-inulin		
0–24 hr	24–96 hr	Total	E109+ (%)	Anti-TNP
Normal Ig[b]	0	26	6	210
Normal Ig	BL	105	37	1838
Normal Ig	NWSM	530	36	2113
Normal Ig	TNP-BA	83	62	2818
Anti-E109	0	35	0	208
Anti-E109	BL	63	0	418
Anti-E109	NWSM	775	2	3815
Anti-E109	TNP-BA	47	0	2100

[a] From Bona et al., 1979b.

[b] 10^7 BALB/c spleen cells were cultured in 35-mm dishes for a total of 96 hours under rocking condition. During the first 24 hours, the cells were cultured with 100 μg/ml of normal A/He immunoglobulin or with 100 μg/ml of A/He anti-E109 immunoglobulin. The cells were washed and cultured for the remainder of the culture period with nothing, BL (10 μg/ml), NWSM (10 μg/ml), or TNP-BA ($\sim$ 100 μg/ml). At the end of this time, the number of anti-inulin PFC and the fraction expressing E109 idiotypes were determined as were the number of anti-TNP-PFC.

tibodies did not alter the stimulating of activity of both TNP-BL and TNP-inulin (Fig. 4.5). These results suggest that idiotype-bearing molecules on B cells specific for defined antigenic determinants on carriers play a critical role in activation of B cells specific for other determinants on the same carrier. In fact, the partial inhibition of the anti-TNP response by anti-E109 and anti-A48 is consistent with the idea that the idiotypes of these two antibodies are carried on distinct families of anti-BL antibody molecules. Therefore the *in vitro* and *in vivo* results showed that anti-Id antibodies can suppress the IdX+ component of a given antibody response by direct interaction of anti-Id antibodies with Id+ receptors of precursors. In addition, clearly, anti-Id antibodies could suppress responses to determinants borne by the same carrier but different from those identified by idiotype-bearing antibody. This indirect suppression was observed in both specific and polyclonal stimulation. The mechanism of this indirect sup-

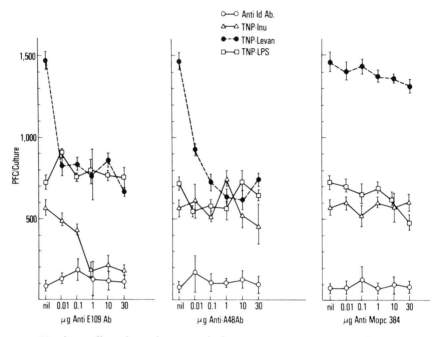

Fig. 4.5. Effect of anti-idiotype antibody on anti-TNP-PFC response after *in vitro* stimulation with TNP-levan, TNP-inulin or *S. tranoroa* LPS-TNP. 10^7 cells were pre-treated for 24 hours with nothing or various amounts of purified anti-E109, anti-A48, or anti-MOPC384 idiotype antibodies. After washing, the cells were recultured for 3 days with nothing, with 0.005 μg TNP -levan, with 10 μg TNP- inulin, or with 25 μg TNP-LPS. Anti-TNP-PFC were measured at the end of the culture period. From Bona *et al.,* 1979c.

pression is not clear. However, it can provide a model for studies of cellular aspects of control of antibody responses by anti-Id sera.

V. Idiotype Suppression Mediated by B Cells (B Cell Dominance)

Eig *et al.* (1977) reported a new phenomenon of idiotype suppression by B dominance. In their experiments, BALB/c mice (H-2^d IgV-h[a] IgC-h[a]) were primed with KLH-phenylarsonate (Ars). B cells from these mice lack IdX controlled by the *IgC-h[d]* genes, but can completely inhibit the appearance of IdX$^+$ anti-Ars antibodies in

C.AL20 (H-2^e IgV-h^e) mice. C.AL20 mice following immunization with KLH-Ars produce IdX$^+$ anti-Ars antibodies. This IdX-bearing anti-Ars antibody response was not inhibited by transfer of normal BALB/c cells or cells from BALB/c mice only immunized with the KLH carrier.

Several hypotheses have been tested to explain this observation.

1. The presence of Id-specific suppressor T cells in BALB/c mice which could exert their effects on the C.AL20 precursor of IdX-bearing anti-Ars cells. In the Ars system the Id-specific T suppressor cells occurred only after administration of anti-Id antibodies (Nisonoff *et al.,* 1977), and their appearance is related to the presence of corresponding *IgC-h* genes (in this case *IgC-h^e*). A decisive experiment which ruled out this explanation was that the pretreatment of spleen cells from BALB/c primed with KLH-Ars with anti-Thy-1.2 plus C did not ablate the suppression of IdX$^+$ anti-Ars response of C.AL20 mice.

2. The same pretreatment excluded another explanation, according to which BALB/c mice, after immunization with KLH-Ars, developed KLH (carrier)-specific suppressor T cells which exerted their effect on CAL.20 carrier-specific helper T cells. In addition, in further experiments spleen cells from BALB/c immunized with BGG-Ars have been transferred in C.AL20 mice which then were immunized with KLH-Ars. In this condition the suppression of IdX$^+$ anti-Ars antibodies was also observed, suggesting clearly that carrier-specific suppressor T cells generated in BALB/c mice cannot be responsible for the B dominance phenomenon.

3. A more likely explanation provided by the authors is the selective capture of antigen by BALB/c memory cells, which prevents the triggering of unprimed cells with receptors of the same specificity. A similar explanation was provided for the dominance of allotype observed in rabbits that recovered from maternally induced allotype suppression (Yamada *et al.,* 1979). The induction of memory cells during early and complete phase of allotype suppression in the young rabbits has been shown to lead to the preferential production of antibodies with nonsuppressed allotype specificity in response to a new antigenic challenge given after spontaneous or induced release from the suppression.

4. Finally, in both experimental systems in which a B dominance has been observed, the participation of B suppressor cells should be taken into consideration. Singhal *et al.* (1978) have shown that such suppres-

sor B cells are present in the murine bone marrow and that they exert their effects during early events of the immune response. In other mammalian species, suppressor B cells have been identified that can alter delayed-type hypersensitivity reactions (Katz *et al.*, 1974) or antigen-specific induced T cell response (Bona *et al.*, 1976; Eyquem and Bona, 1977).

VI. *In Vitro* Idiotypic Suppression of Secretion of Ig by Leukemic Cells

Most patients with chronic lymphocytic leukemia (CLL) manifest a monoclonal proliferation of B cells, and therefore the majority of leukemic lymphocytes express the same Id determinants on their sIg. However, frequently there is a defect in the ability of leukemic cells to differentiate into plasma cells. This maturational defect is variable, and

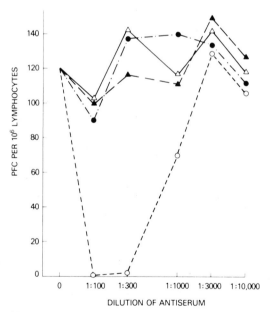

Fig. 4.6. Effect of various dilutions of antisera on the spontaneous (day 0) anti-SRBC PFC response of the patient's lymphocytes. Only the sheep anti-Id suppressed spontaneous anti-SRBC PFC responses. ●, sheep preimmunization; ○, sheep anti-Id; ▲, guinea pig preimmunization; △, guinea pig anti-Id. From Bona and Fauci, 1980.

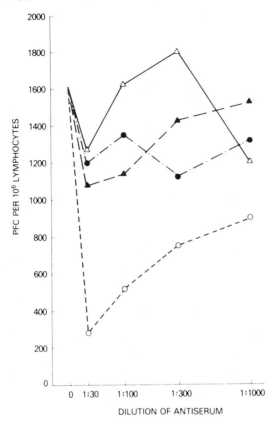

Fig. 4.7. Effect of various antisera on the PWM-induced anti-SRBC PFC response of the patient's lymphocytes. The antisera were added to cultures on day 0 together with PWM, and anti-SRBC PFC responses were measured after 6 days of culture. Only the sheep anti-Id antiserum suppressed the anti-SRBC PFC responses. ●, sheep preimmunization; ○, sheep anti-Id; ▲, guinea pig preimmunization; △, guinea pig anti-Id. From Bona and Fauci, 1980.

in some cases the B cells from leukemic patients secrete Ig. We have studied a patient with CLL who had a monoclonal IgM band that bound SRBC. An anti-Id serum was obtained in a sheep by immunization with autologous erythrocytes that were previously coated with the monoclonal IgM anti-SRBC antibodies. The monoclonal anti-SRBC antibodies in the serum and on the surface of the patient's B cells were shown to be idiotypically identical. In addition, the peripheral blood lymphocytes from this patient showed more than

100 spontaneous anti-SRBC PFC/10^6. The sheep anti-Id antibodies suppressed the spontaneous anti-SRBC PFC response at dilutions of 1 : 100 to 1 : 300 and suppressed to almost 50% of control at dilution of 1 : 100 (Fig. 4.6). The effects of anti-Id serum have been tested on PWM-induced anti-SRBC PFC. Anti-id antibodies markedly suppressed the PWM-induced anti-SRBC PFC response of the CLL patient's lymphocytes, whereas they did not affect the response of lymphocytes from several normal volunteers (Fig. 4.7). The suppression was less dramatic than that of the spontaneously secreting B cells, but it was nonetheless profound (Bona and Fauci, 1980). The suppression induced by anti-Id antibodies was not overcome by a powerful stimulus such as polyclonal B-cell mitogen as PWM. This is of interest in that other findings showed that allotype suppression or tolerance induced by antigens can be broken by B cell mitogens (Fernandez *et al.*, 1979; Bona *et al.*, 1977; Weigle, and Parks, 1978).

This study clearly demonstrated that the leukemic cells are susceptible to immunoregulatory signals and that anti-Id antibodies can interact with Id$^+$ sIg of leukemic cells and inhibit the antibody secretion.

VII. Inhibition of Growth of Myeloma Cells by Anti-idiotypic Antibodies

After the discovery of Sirisinha and Eisen (1971) that anti-Id antibodies can be obtained in syngeneic systems, several authors took advantage of this observation to study the effects of anti-idiotypic immunity on the growth of myeloma cells. One year after that observation was made, Lynch *et al.* (1972) showed that BALB/c mice immunized with two myeloma proteins (i.e., MOPC315 and MOPC460) and which produced anti-315Id and anti-460Id antibodies, respectively, failed to develop tumors when they were grafted with MOPC315 and MOPC460 tumor cells. The resistance to myeloma cells was idiotype-specific, since mice rendered resistant to MOPC315 were not significantly resistant to MOPC460-grafted cells. Eisen *et al.* (1975) considered that Id determinants expressed on sIg of myeloma cells behave as tumor-specific transplantation antigens and that they could be the targets of various immune regulatory effects. The inhibition of growth of myeloma cells after immunization with the corresponding myeloma proteins was obtained by various investigators

(Meinke *et al.*, 1974; Freedman *et al.*, 1976). A similar effect of anti-Id antibodies was observed in the case of lymphoma. Sugai *et al.* (1974) prepared anti-Id antibodies against monoclonal IgM produced by the 141 lymphoma tumor (which can also occur spontaneously in B/W strain of mice). The majority of lymphoma cells in this case carry Id^+ sIgM. Immunization of B/W mice with 141 IgM monoclonal protein before the transplantation of lymphoma cells confers resistance against lymphoma cells. Haughton *et al.* (1978) obtained anti-Id antibodies against IgM of CH_1 B cell lymphoma. Interestingly, in this study the protection against lymphoma cells was observed even when the anti-Id serum was administered 2 days after the graft of CH_1 tumor. Therefore, it appears that the growth of myeloma or lymphoma does not represent an autonomous malignant process which is not susceptible to any immunoregulatory signals. This was clearly shown in the experiments of Lynch *et al.* (1979) which studied the growth and differentiation of MOPC315 cells in Millipore diffusion chambers implanted into the peritoneal cavity of BALB/c mice. In this experimental system they studied the effects of helper and suppressor cells specific for SRBC in the presence of SRBC-TNP which is bound to the receptors of MOPC315 cells. SRBC-specific helper T cells enhanced, whereas SRBC-specific suppressor T cells inhibited, their growth. If the anti-Id antibodies by themselves are responsible for the idiotype-specific graft resistance, we should ask why the mice injected with myeloma cells which secrete Id^+ monoclonal proteins which are immunogenic in a syngeneic system cannot elicit a protective Id-specific immunity. In fact, anti-Id antibodies or Id–anti-Id complexes were never detected in the sera of mice bearing myeloma tumors. However, Serban *et al.* (1979) have found in the mice with MOPC460 or MOPC315 myeloma tumors lymphocytes and plasma cells which rosetted SRBC coated with MOPC460 or MOPC315 myeloma proteins. The precursor of these cells certainly exists in the normal BALB/c mice and can be activated in anti-460Id producing cells after immunization with MOPC460 myeloma protein (Bona *et al.*, 1979a).

These results suggest that 460Id or 315Id specific cells are generated during the development of myeloma tumor, but probably their products are rapidly neutralized by Id^+ monoclonal antibodies. Since the anti-Id antibodies were detected neither in the serum nor on the surface of lymphocytes and no Id–anti-Id complexes were identified, it appears that anti-Id-forming cells do not play a major role in the Id-specific resistance against myeloma cells. By contrast, regulatory T cells could play a role. In an elegant study Daley *et al.* (1978) have shown that the idiotype-specific immunity for MOPC315 myeloma cells can be abrogated by adult thymectomy. These findings indicate that anti-idiotypic antibodies can represent a potential therapeutic tool to manage the growth of myeloma.

5

Idiotypic Determinants and T Cells

I. Introduction

Thymus-derived (T) lymphocyte population is constituted from various subsets which possess different immunological functions and express particular antigens. T cells bear on their membrane cytodifferentiation antigens characteristic for each mammalian species (e.g. murine Thy, rabbit RTLA, and human HTLA) as well as receptors for nonspecific lectin mitogens.

Three major subsets constitute the T cell population.

a. Effector T cells which mediate cellular immune responses, such as antigen-specific induced blast proliferation, delayed-type hypersensitivity, graft versus host reactions, rejection of allo- and heterografts, and cell-specific cytotoxicity. Some of these effector cells express Ia and Lyt antigens.

b. Helper T cells which deliver stimulatory signals for the activation of B cells by T-dependent antigens. These cells express Lyt 1 antigens but lack Ia determinants.

c. Suppressor T cells which play a regulatory role on the humoral and cell-mediated immune response and can exert their effects on helper T cells, effector T cells, or B cells. They express Lyt 2.3 and I-J antigens.

These three subsets of T lymphocytes have an antigen-specific receptor which does not bear the antigenic determinants of constant region of Ig molecules. Numerous data accumulated in the past 5 years have shown that the antigenic receptors of T cells express Id determinants of humoral antibodies.

This demonstration has two major implications which indicate that the same set of V genes controls the specificity of antigen-specific T and B cells and that the Id determinants borne by T cells might serve as sites of regulatory effects of anti-Id antibodies.

II. V Region Expressed on the Antigen-Binding Receptor of T Cells

The discovery of idiotypy has contributed to the understanding of the mechanism of generation of diversity of antibody and to the organization of variable of antibody molecules responsible for the antigen specificity. The role of idiotype in the physiology of the immune system came to be understood when Id determinants were identified on antigen-binding receptors of B and T cells.

The presence of antigen-binding receptors on T cells was largely documented during the early 1970s, indicating that T cells recognize conventional and alloantigens (Benacerraf and McDevitt, 1972). Later, it was shown that T cells can recognize antigens only in the presence of self-antigens encoded by MHC. Thus, the cyolytic T cells specific for hapten self-target recognize the antigen and self-H-2 antigens (Shearer et al., 1976), while helper T cells and effector T cells of delayed-type hypersensitivity reaction might see Ia self-antigens (Katz et al., 1975; Vadas et al., 1976). However, the majority of the investigators failed to find the antigenic determinants of Ig receptors of B cells on the T cells (Crone et al., 1972; Lisowska-Bernstein et al., 1973; Vitetta et al., 1973).

Therefore, the discovery of Id determinants on the receptors of T cells gave a new insight on the mechanisms which govern the specificity in the immune system. The discovery of Id determinants on the antigen-binding receptors of T and B cells, as well as that the anti-Id antibodies possess regulatory functions, led to the concept that Id determinants might serve as sites for the physiological regulation of lymphocyte functions.

The first breakthrough which permitted the study of Id determinants on the T cells was performed by the preparation of anti-Id sera which interacted with the receptor of T cells.

These anti-idiotypic sera were prepared initially by (a) immunization of F_1 hybrids with alloantisera obtained from animals injected with allogenic cells (Ramseier and Lindemann, 1971) or grafted with allogenic skin (Binz and Lindemann, 1972) and (b) immunization of F_1 with parental T cells (Ramseier, 1973) or with T cell receptor shed in the culture medium (Ramseier and Lindemann 1972).

These anti-Id sera bound to alloantigen-binding receptors of lymphocytes, and this binding was inhibited by alloantibodies. However, the findings obtained between 1971 and 1973 did not show clearly that anti-Id antibodies interacted with T cells.

The staining of Id determinants on the receptors of T cells by Binz *et al.* (1974) and their demonstration in functional experiments by Eichmann (1974) drew great interest, and it was suggested that the same set of *V* genes controls the specificity of antigen-binding receptors of B and T cells.

A. Idiotypic Determinants Expressed on Antigen-Binding T Cells

The presence of Id determinants on antigen-binding cells (ABC) was studied in various antigenic systems and mammalian species. The results of these observations can be divided into two groups with regard to the specificity of the receptors of T cells to bind the allo- and foreign antigens.

1. Alloreactive T Cells

Indications that T and B cells reactive to alloantigens share Id determinants came from early studies of Ramseier and Lindemann (1971) and Binz and Wigzell (1975a). However, the anti-Id antisera obtained by this time had been too weak to permit a direct observation of Id determinants on T cells. This became possible only after the conditions of preparation of anti-Id antibodies were optimized. Binz and Wigzell (1975a) prepared anti-Id sera by immunization of F_1 hybrids with purified T lymphocytes from one of the parental strains. These anti-Id antibodies were equally removed by adsorption on T cells and alloantibody immunoadsorbants. These anti-Id antibodies have been used for direct observation of cells bearing Id determinants and to determine the frequency of T and B cells which shared the idiotypes of alloantibodies. This study was performed on Lewis rats with anti-Id antibodies specific for Lewis anti-DA alloantibodies.

The frequency of T lymphocytes bearing Id determinants of anti-DA specificity was 6.2%, whereas of B cells only 1.1%. Similar results were obtained with fluoresceinated anti-Id antibodies by immuno-fluorescence and with iodine-labeled antibodies by autoradiography. The relatively high frequency of T cells bearing allo-specific receptors observed in this study matched with earlier findings using entirely different approaches. This high frequency can be related to the ability of anti-Id antibodies to interact with multiple idiotypes and not with a unique Id determinant expressed on the receptors of T cells. The cytofluorospectrophotometry measurements indicated a high density of Id^+ receptors on the surface of T and B cells (Binz and Wigzell, 1975c). In further experiments, Binz and Wigzell (1975b) have shown that Id^+ T cells can be separated from T cells lacking Id determinants via incubation of T cells with beads coated with an IgG fraction of anti-Id antibodies.

This approach provided a useful means to study the immunoreactivity of these cells. The T cells enriched in Id^+ cells retained their full capacity to cause graft versus host (GVH) reaction, while the cells preparations depleted of Id^+ cells failed to provoke GVH reaction. A striking, positive correlation was found between the percentage of Lewis anti-DA Id^+ T cells and the anti-DA-GVH reaction. These findings indicated that the B and T cells reactive to alloantigens shared Id determinants and that it was possible to use anti-Id antibodies to enumerate the alloreactive lymphocytes in both T and B compartments.

Krammer (1978) provided direct evidence that Id determinants are expressed on the alloantigen-binding receptors of T cells. He prepared anti-Id antibodies in F_1 (AKR $\times$ C57BL/6) hybrids by immunization with AKR T blasts obtained in MLC with C57BL/6 stimulating cells. These anti-Id antibodies were removed by passage over an IgG fraction of anti-C57BL/6 alloantibody immunoadsorbant.

The binding of fluoresceinated anti-Id antibodies to AKR anti-B6 T blasts was inhibited by B6 membrane preparations. These results indicated that Id determinants are carried on the alloantigen-binding receptors of T cells. Interestingly, the anti-Id antibodies stained the same number of anti-B6-AKR of F_1 (AKR $\times$ SJL) T blasts. These results excluded the existence of an IdX on the B6-specific antigen receptors of AKR and SJL. However, the fact that the same percentage of T blasts of AKR and (AKR × SJL)F_1 were stained by anti-Id antibodies suggests the absence of allelic exclusion at T cell receptor levels. If this is true, a fundamental difference exists between the receptors of T cell and B cell, since this later shows allelic exclusion.

The presence of Id determinants on alloantigen-reactive T cells was also reported by Rubin *et al.* (1979). In this study, an anti-Id antiserum prepared in rabbit following immunization with C57BL/6 anti-CBA alloantibodies was used. After adequate adsorptions it was shown that this anti-Id antiserum reacted only with anti-H-2^b antibodies and with H-2^b-reactive T cells.

Interestingly, by using various congenic strains of mice, Rubin *et al.* (1979) have found that anti-Id antibodies were directed particularly against receptors specific for I-A^k alloantigens.

In summary, these data clearly demonstrated that the receptors of T cells reactive to alloantigens share the idiotypic determinants of alloantibodies as well as of allo-reactive B cells.

2. T Cells Reactive to Foreign Antigens

The majority of the reported findings agree that antigen-binding receptors of T cells do not express the antigenic determinants of constant region of Ig molecules. However, the receptors of T cells discriminate with great precision between closely related antigenic determinants and recognize the haptens as well as the carriers (Janneway *et al.*, 1977).

As the receptor of T cells reactive to alloantigens, the receptor of T cells reactive to foreign antigens express antigenic determinants of the *V* region.

At least three or four series of antigenic determinants have been localized within the *V* region: (1) idiotypic determinants associated with combining site or framework segments probably yielding anti-Id antibodies; (2) framework segments which determine the subgroup assignment of the *V* region; (3) so-called *V*-domain-specific antigens probably yielding the anti- V_H and V_L antibodies; and (4) in some species, the allotype of V_H region as *a* series allotype in rabbit or their U10-173 equivalent in mice. Some of these antigenic determinants have been identified on the antigen-binding receptor of T cells.

Lonai *et al.* (1978) studied the antigen-binding cells (ABC) in normal and immunized C3H-SW mice with (T,G)-A--L synthetic antigen. They observed that both subsets of T lymphocytes having Lyt 1^+ or Lyt 2^+3^+ phenotype contain T cells which bind (T,G) A--L antigen.

The number of ABC T cells was increased in short-term cultures when Lyt 1^+-selected T cells were cultured with a soluble macrophage factor and when Lyt 2^+3^+-selected T cells were cultured with mouse viral interferon. By using this method the number of ABC was considerably enriched and therefore the effects of various antisera have been easily studied.

The effects of anti-Id, anti-allotypic, and anti-V_H and -V_L, anti-Ia, and anti-H-2 antisera were studied on the antigen-binding capacity of T cells originating from normal and immune mice.

Anti-Id antibodies inhibited equally the ABC from normal and immune C3H-SW mice. This inhibition was specific since it did not affect the binding of an irrelevant antigen (i.e., TEPC15). In addition, the anti-Id antibodies against C3H-SW anti-(T,G)-A--L antibodies did not inhibit the ABC from CWB congenic mice (which bear a different allotype). Anti-allotype antibodies had no inhibitory effect on ABC T cells, but they inhibited the ABC-B cells.

Anti-V_H serum (goat anti-Fv fragments of MOPC315) inhibited Lyt 1^+ ABC-T cells from normal and immune mice and had a little inhibitory effect on B cells. Anti-V_L serum inhibited Lyt 2^+3^+ ABC T cells, but had no effect on immune ABC T cells.

Finally, anti-Ia antibodies inhibited Lyt 1^+ ABC T cells, whereas anti-H-2 antibodies inhibited the cells bearing Lyt 2^+3^+ antigens. These results indicated that the ABC T cells from normal and immune animals expressed Id determinants but that the framework determinants are selectively expressed on various subsets of lymphocytes, despite the fact that they have the same antigen-binding activity. It appears that there is a fundamental difference between the receptor of T cells and B cells. A T cell receptor expresses one or the other V-chain determinant but never both.

From this study it did not appear clear whether or not antigen-binding receptor of T cells belongs to a complex which contains H-2 and Ia antigens encoded by MHC. Indeed, the inhibition of ABC T cells by anti-H-2 or Ia antisera can be due to a hindrance.

Id determinants were also identified on the receptor of rabbit T cells together with other markers of V region. The rabbit represents a unique model to study the expression of various antigenic determinants of V region, since a series allotype in this species are located on V_H region of Ig molecules. We studied the presence of various V_H markers on RNase-binding T cells from immune rabbits by using three antisera: (1) homologous anti-Id sera directed against rabbit anti-bovine RNase; (2) homologous anti-*a* series allotype antisera; and (3) goat anti-rabbit V_H antisera.

Rabbit T cells were prepared according to the method of Cavaillon *et al.* (1977). The degree of the purification of the T cells was controlled by various techniques. These cells were killed with anti-RTLA serum and complement (C) and developed a vigorous proliferative response to concanavalin A (Con A). By contrast, they were not stimulated by NWSM, were not killed by anti-RABELA serum + C, and were not stained by anti-rabbit Ig antibodies. Details of these techniques and the interpretation of these results have been reviewed elsewhere (Bona *et al.*, 1977).

The Id-bearing T cells were visualized by staining with peroxidase-labeled $F(ab')_2$ anti-Id antibodies and by Id-RFC method. In this assay, lymphocytes bearing Id^+ receptors and SRBC coated with Fab fragment of anti-RNase antibodies were cross-linked with $F(ab')_2$ fragment of anti-Id antibodies (Fig. 5.1).

The percentage of cells binding RNase varied from 1.3 to 4.2% and of Id rosette-forming cells (RFC) from 1.8 to 5.7%. The specificity of Id RFC method was demonstrated by the low number of Id-RFC when lymphocytes from normal rabbits were used, the absence of Id-RFC when a "wrong" anti-Id antibody was used, and strong inhibition of Id

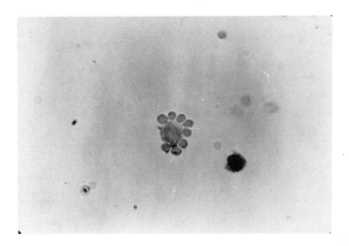

Fig. 5.1.   Idiotype rosette forming cells. RNase-coated SRBC were sensitized with Id bearing anti-RNase antibodies and then incubated with lymphocytes and anti-Id antibodies.

RFC when the lymphocytes have been preincubated with the corresponding anti-Id antibodies (Table 5.1).

Unseparated, B and T purified lymphocytes bound ^{125}I-labeled anti-Id antibodies. The amount of radioactivity bound to lymphocytes was dependent on the number of cells. At higher concentration of cells (10^6), the B cells bound more radioactive anti-Id antibodies than the T cells (Fig. 5.2). Enumeration of Id$^+$ T cells after the staining with peroxidase-labeled antibodies or by Id-RFC method indicated that from 1.2 to 1.7% of T cells bore Id determinants of anti-RNase antibodies (Table 5.2).

The expression of various antigenic determinants of Ig molecules on the receptor of Ig$^+$ and Ig$^-$ cells was studied on the lymphocytes from a single rabbit. The same percentage of Ig$^+$ cells was stained with anti-Ig, anti-b4, and anti-a1 antisera (i.e., 80–86%), whereas anti-V_H stained only 38% and anti-Id antibodies 3.8% of the B cells. By

TABLE 5.1

Percentage of Lymphocytes Carrying Idiotypic Determinants Estimated by Mixed Agglutination (Id-RFC)[a]

Rabbit number donor of lymphocytes	Rabbit number donor of anti-RNase Ab used to coat SRBC	Anti-idiotypic Ab	% RNase binding cells	% of Id-RFC	% of inhibition of Id-RFC with anti-Id-Ab[c]
969	969	anti-969	2.9	3.9	80
695	695	anti-695	1.3	1.8	70
440	440	anti-440	1.6	3.8	ND[e]
881	881	anti-881	1.6	2.5	98
882	882	anti-881[d]	4.7	5.7	93
886	886	anti-881	1.9	0.9	60
1[b]	881	anti-881	0.5	0.4	ND
2[b]	969	anti-969	0.2	0	—

[a] From Cazenave *et al.,* 1977a.

[b] Nonimmunized rabbits.

[c] SRBC coated with RNase and anti-RNase Ab were incubated for 30 minutes with anti-idiotypic antibody before being incubated with lymphocytes.

[d] Anti-881 idiotypic serum cross-reacted with RNase antibodies of rabbit 882.

[e] ND, not done.

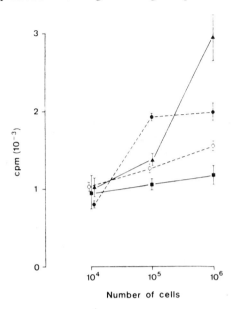

Fig. 5.2. Binding of ^{125}I-labeled F(ab')$_2$ fragments of anti-idiotypic antibody (anti-695). ■—■, nonseparated lymphocytes from a nonimmunized rabbit; ○—○, nonseparated lymphocytes from RNase immunized rabbit (No. 695); ▲—▲, B lymphocytes from rabbit 695; ●—●, T lymphocytes from rabbit 695.

TABLE 5.2

Percentage of Cells Carrying Idiotypic Markers[a,b]

Rabbit number donor of lymphocytes	Anti-idiotypic antibody	Nonseparated lymphocytes		T-derived lymphocytes	
		% Id-RFC	% cells stained	% Id-RFC	% cells stained
695	anti-695	1.75	1.80	1.35	1.33
440	anti-440	1.0	3.8	1.69	6.81
969	anti-969	3.9	3.59	1.2	1.61

[a] From Cazenave *et al.,* 1977a.

[b] Estimated by mixed agglutination technique and staining with peroxidase-labeled F(ab')$_2$ fragments of anti-idiotypic antibody. Comparison between nonseparated lymphocytes and T-derived lymphocytes.

contrast, the percentage of Ig$^-$ cells stained with anti-Ig and anti-b4 was very low. Anti-V$_H$ serum stained 18%, anti-a1 13.3%, and anti-Id 6.8% of T cells (Table 5.3).

Interestingly, T cells from normal rabbits have not been stained by anti-a allotype antibodies, indicating that the immunization could increase the density of the receptors of T cells.

Supporting evidence of the V origin on the receptor of T cells comes from the study of distribution of idiotypes, a-series allotypes, and V$_H$ framework determinants on Id-RFC T cells. Positively selected Id$^+$ T cells by Id-RFC method were not stained with anti-rabbit Ig and anti-b4 allotype antibodies. More than 30% were stained by anti-Id and anti-V$_H$ antibodies and 60% by anti-a- series allotype antibodies (Table 5.4) (Cazenave *et al.*, 1977).

Our results have been confirmed by Krawinkel *et al.* (1977). In this study the authors isolated hapten-binding receptors from Ig$^+$ and Ig$^-$ rabbit lymphocytes. The receptor of Ig$^+$ cells was retained on immunoadsorbants made with anti-Ig class-specific antibodies, as well as H and K chains. The receptor of Ig$^-$ rabbit lymphocytes was retained on anti-a allotype antibodies immunoadsorbant.

These results taken collectively shown that in rabbits, as in mice, the antigen-binding receptor of T cells expressed Id determinants, as well as other phenotypic markers of V_H region. However, it should be mentioned that according to our studies T cells bearing Id$^+$ receptors

TABLE 5.3

Percentage of Nonseparated T (Ig$^-$) and B (Ig$^+$)-Derived Lymphocytes Stained with Peroxidase-Labeled F(ab')$_2$ Fragments of Several Antibodies[a]

Source of peroxidase-labeled F(ab')$_2$ fragments	Nonseparated lymphocytes (%)	Ig$^+$ lymphocytes (%)	Ig$^-$ lymphocytes[b] (%)
Goat anti-rabbit Ig antibody	30	82	4.56
Rabbit anti-b4 anti-allotypic antibody	36.67	80.6	4.69
Rabbit anti-a$_1$ anti-allotypic antibody	38.64	86	13.3
Anti-440 anti-idiotypic antibody	3.8	8.9	6.81
Goat anti-rabbit V$_H$ antibody	36.36	38	18

[a] In these experiments the lymphocytes originated from rabbit 440 [phenotype a(1$^+$2$^-$3$^-$) b(4$^+$5$^-$6$^-$)].

[b] 70.89% of this population was killed by anti-RTLA serum and 3% with anti-RABELA serum (source of complement: b9/b9 homozygous rabbit).

TABLE 5.4

Percentage of Id-RFC Formed by Ig⁻ Cells Stained with Peroxidase-Labeled F(ab′)₂ Fragments of Goat Anti-Rabbit Ig, Anti-V_H, of Rabbit Anti-a1, Anti-b4, and Anti-Id Antibodies

Source of peroxidase-labeled F(ab′)₂ fragments	Id-RFC stained (%)
Goat anti-rabbit Ig antibody	0
Rabbit anti-b4 antibody	0
Rabbit anti-a1 antibody	65
Rabbit anti-Id antibody	92
Goat anti-rabbit V_H antibody	93

can be divided into a⁺ and a⁻ subsets. It is not clear why the *a* allotype can be detected only in immunized rabbits and only on a fraction of Id⁺ T cells.

The presence of Id determinants on the surface of guinea pig T cells was studied by Prange *et al.* (1977) following immunization with L-tyrosine-L-azophenyltrimethylammonium (TMA). The antigen-binding cells were scored in autoradiography using ¹²⁵I-BSA-TMA. A specific anti-Id antibody has been prepared in rabbit immunized with purified guinea pig anti-TMA antibodies. The presence of Id determinants on antigen-binding receptor was studied on separated Ig⁺ and Ig⁻ cells. Anti-Ig class-specific antibodies inhibited 90–100%. The ABC T cells were inhibited 80% by anti-Id antibodies but not by anti-Ig antibodies.

The T cells recovered antigen-binding capacity inhibitable by anti-Id antibodies subsequent to trypsin treatment after 16 hours of culture. These results indicated that the receptor of T cells was of endogenous origin.

Interestingly, the antigen-binding capacity of T cells was also inhibited by two anti-strain 13 anti-Ia sera, which suggests a possible association of Ia antigen with antigen receptor of T cells. The existence of Id determinants on the human T cells was demonstrated only in the subjects with myeloma.

Preud'homme *et al.* (1977) studied the presence of Id determinants of a myeloma protein of horse 2M-binding activity on the surface of T and B lymphocytes. Anti-Id antibodies have been prepared in rabbits. Fluoresceinated anti-Id antibodies stained 25–30% of the peripheral blood lymphocytes and 4.3% of T cells selected by their ability to form rosettes with SRBC. The idiotypic determinants expressed on the receptor of T cells were not cytophilic antibodies, since they were regenerated after the trypsin treatment.

Similar results were obtained by Lea *et al.* (1979) in a patient with an IgA monoclonal protein with anti-streptolysin O activity. Between 5 and 8% of T lymphocyte-enriched population of the patient bound streptolysin O antigen, as well as were stained with $F(ab')_2$ fragments of anti-Id antibodies.

It should be mentioned that in other patients with myeloma or with chronic lymphoid leukemia, the anti-Id antibodies prepared against monoclonal proteins did not interact with the T cells from these patients (Kubagawa *et al.*, 1979; Bona and Fauci, 1980). No explanations exist for this discrepancy. However, these results indicate that the Id determinants are expressed on the receptor of T cells reactive for allo- and foreign antigens.

3. Control of Idiotypes of T Cell Receptor by Genes of Heavy Chain Linkage Group

It was shown in several antigenic systems that the expression of *V* genes which encode the idiotypic specificities is under the control of *C-h* genes. In these cases the Id determinants and the allotypes segregate together (see Chapter 1). There is suggestive evidence indicating that this rule also governs the expression of Id determinants on the receptor of T cells.

Binz *et al.* (1976) have studied the relationship between the expression of Id determinants of Lewis anti-DA-reactive T cells and the presence of Lewis IgA and *k*-chain allotypes.

They studied eight F_2 individuals (Lewis × DA) hybrids for the presence of Lewis allotype, idiotypes of Lewis anti-DA T cells, and the response in MLC of the cells stimulated against DA- and BN-stimulating cells.

Three rats which were homozygous for DA heavy chain failed to express the Id determinants, whereas the other five having Lewis IgA allotype markers expressed the idiotypes of Lewis anti-DA-specific T cells. Similar results were obtained by Krammer (1978) who showed that the expression of Id of receptor of T cell blasts activated in MLC is under the control of *C-h* genes.

In these experiments an anti-Id serum prepared in F_1 (C57BL/6 ×

AKR) against AKR anti-B6 T blasts was used. This anti-Id serum did not react with SJL anti-B6 T blasts. AKR mice are of H-2^k and Ig-1^d type, and SJL mice of H-2^s and Ig-1^b type. The expression of Id determinants was studied in the progeny from backcross (AKR × SJL) × SJL. Only the hybrids of H-2$^{s/k}$ and Ig-1$^{b/d}$ expressed the Id determinants of AKR T cells specific for H-2^b alloantigens.

Rubin *et al.* (1979) studied the distribution of Id determinants expressed on C57BL/6 T blasts specific for H-2^k alloantigens in various strains of mice. This idiotype was found only on T cells originating from mice bearing Ig-1^b and Ig-1^b but not Ig-1^a allotype. In these experiments rabbit anti-Id serum prepared against C57BL/6 anti-CBA alloantibodies was used. This can explain the results that expression of Id determinants of C57BL/6 T blasts specific for H-2^k alloantigens was found not only in the mice bearing *Ig-1^b* allotype but also in *Ig-1^c*. These data are in agreement with previous observations which showed that expression of Id determinants on helper and suppressor T cells is linked to *Ig-1* genes.

Hammerling and Eichmann (1976) reported that guinea pig anti-A5A Id antibodies reacted with A-CHO-specific helper T cells. This reaction was restricted to strains of mice bearing *Ig-1^c* allotype.

Recently, we have shown that BALB/c mice have naturally occurring 460Id-specific suppressor T cells which regulate the expression of clones secreting 460Id$^+$ anti-TNP antibodies (Bona and Paul, 1979a). The activity of these cells can be enhanced by immunization of BALB/c mice with MOPC460 myeloma proteins (Bona and Paul, 1979a). We have found that 460Id in anti-TNP antibodies developed in both BALB/c and C58/J mice which both possess *V-h* and *C-h* genes of BALB/c mice, whereas other BALB/c congenic strains of mice which lack BALB/c *C-h* genes failed to express 460Id. We have studied the occurrence of 460Id-specific suppressor T cells in several strains of mice.

C.B20—a BALB/c congenic strain which has *V-h* and *C-h* genes of C57BL/Ka mice (Ig-1^b)

C.AL20—a BALB/c congenic strain which has *V-h* and *C-h* genes of AL.N mice (Ig-1^c)

C58/J—a strain of H-2^k type which has *Igh-C^a* genes and at least some *V-h* genes similar to BALB/c mice

BAB.14—a BALB/c congenic strain which has *V-h* genes of BALB/c and had *C-h* genes of C57BL/Ka

The 460Id-specific suppressor T cells were identified only in the strains of mice which are of Igh-C^a types.

Since these 460Id-specific suppressor T cells share Id determinants of anti-460Id antibodies (Bona *et al.*, 1979c) we can conclude that the expression of Id determinants on antigen-binding receptor of T cells as well as on idiotype-binding receptor of T cells can be under the control of *C-h* genes.

The control by *Ig* genes may be indirect in that such cells may expand as the result of exposure to B cell products which bear corresponding allotype markers.

B. Idiotypic Determinants Expressed on the Isolated Receptor of T Cells

The isolation of the receptor of T cells and the study of its immune reactivity and biological properties represented an important step in the understanding of function of genes which encode the antigen-binding specificities.

Binz and Wigzell (1974d) have observed that the sera and the urine of normal Lewis rats each contain naturally occurring molecules reactive to allogenic Ag-B antigens. In this study two families of molecules have been identified: one of 7 S in size and the other of 35,000 MW, as was shown by their profile after filtration on Sephadex G-200.

Both molecules bound to DA-alloantigens and expressed Id determinants of Lewis anti-DA alloantibodies. These molecules were removed after the adsorption over anti-Id antibody immunoadsorbant, and they were able to elicit the production of anti-Id antibodies in rabbits or in chickens. These kinds of molecules were also purified from the fluid of the cultures of T and B cells. From B cell cultures there was obtained 7 S types of molecules, whereas from T cell culture the low molecular weight molecules were obtained (Binz and Wigzell, 1975d). The SDS polyacrylamide electrophoresis analysis of these molecules externally (with ^{125}I) or internally (with ^{3}H) labeled indicated that the molecules secreted by B cells are 7 S to 8 S IgM. The molecules shed off by T cells had 150,000 MW consisting of two similar chains. These molecules can be easily degradated into 35,000 MW components by serum factors (Binz *et al.*, 1976). The T cell product which interacted with anti-Id antibodies failed to react with antisera specific for constant region antigenic determinants of Ig molecule as well as with anti-Ag-B antibodies. These results indicated that T cell receptor is constituted solely by two V_H region polypeptide chains.

The T receptorlike material was purified and isolated on anti-Id antibody immunoadsorbants. The immunoreactivity of these purified T receptors was studied with regard to their ability to bind purified antigens encoded by MHC. These antigens were obtained from three strains of rats (DA, BN, and Lewis) LPS blasts. In this experiment the ability of Lewis anti-DA-T cell receptor to bind purified allo- and self-MHC antigens was studied (Binz *et al.,* 1979b). The results of these experiments have shown that Lewis anti-DA-T cell receptors (a) were able to bind to DA-Ag-B and Ia heavy chains but not to the light chain of DA-Ia type, (b) had a significant affinity for self-Ia heavy chain, and (c) failed to bind BN MHC chains (control of the experiment). These important results suggest that allogenic reactive T cells recognize allo- and self-Ia heavy chains and heavy chains of Ag-B antigens.

The molecular size and the structure of the receptor of human T cells was studied on T cells originating from two patients with myeloma. As we mentioned above, a high percentage of T lymphocytes from these two patients shared Id determinants of myeloma proteins.

The results of SDS gel electrophoresis analysis of internally labeled receptor indicate that two families of molecules bore Id determinants: one of 150,000 MW which corresponds to IgG, and another of 140,000 MW which is a dimer of 72,000 MW-type of molecule (Prud'homme *et al.,* 1977; Lea *et al.,* 1979). These results are consistent with those obtained by Binz *et al.* (1976) in rats.

An important step in the study of the expression of various *V* region markers on the receptor of T cells was made by the development of a technique to purify and isolate the antigen-binding receptor of T cells. This technique has as a principle the adherence at 4° C of antigen-specific T or B cells to nylon wool coupled with antigen followed by a temperature shift to remove the cells. The receptor of cells adhering to antigen nylon mesh is then eluted and its activity tested in a highly sensitive phage-inactivation technique (Krawinkel *et al.,* 1977). This technique was used to isolate the receptor from C57BL/6 mouse lymphocytes immunized with 4-hydroxy-3-nitrophenyl acetate (NP). These mice manifested a restricted antibody response to NP and then made antibodies having a high affinity for NIP-related hapten. This type of antibody response was called heteroclitic. The majority of these heteroclitic antibodies carries NP-idiotype which is under the control of *Ig-1^b* genes (Mäkelä *et al.,* 1977). The receptor isolated from C57BL/6 mice consisted of two families: one which reacted with anti-Ig antibodies (Ig$^+$) and which is of B cell origin, and the other which did not react with anti-Ig antibodies (Ig$^-$) of T cell origin. The Ig$^-$ NP-binding receptors expressed Id determinants of anti-NP antibodies, since 74% of their inhibitory activity in phage technique was removed by anti-NP Id antibody immunoadsorbants. The Ig$^-$ NP-binding receptor represents a product of T cells. This was clearly demonstrated by Krawinkel *et al.* (1978) in experiments performed in nude mice chimeras. These were obtained by injection of CB20 T cells in nude BALB/c mice. CB20 mice are congenic with BALB/c mice but possess Ig and Igh-C of b type, whereas BALB/c mice are Ig-1^a type. The BALB/c mice failed to express NP^{b}Id which is Ig-1^b linked. However, the Ig$^-$ NP-binding receptor of these nude mice chimeras expressed NP^b idiotype. This experiment clearly showed the endogenous origin of NP-receptor of T cells. Cramer *et al.* (1979) have found that the V-h framework but not V-1 framework determinants are also expressed on NP-binding receptor of T cells. Taken together, these results indicate that various antigenic markers are expressed on the antigen-binding receptor of T cells.

The discovery of *V* region markers on the receptor on T cells and the immunochemical characterization of the properties of these receptors has had several implications, as follows: (1) indicated that the same set of *V* genes controls the specificity of the receptor of T and B cells; (2) suggested that idiotype restriction can play an important role in the cooperation between T and B cells in the immune response, since the idiotypes represent one of the self-component recognized within immune systems; and (3) suggested that the Id determinants of the receptor of T cells might serve as sites for the regulation of the immune response by anti-Id antibodies.

III. Idiotypic Determinants on the Effector T Cells

The effector T cells represent a heterogenous population of lymphocytes which mediate a variety of cellular immune responses, such as cytotoxic, delayed-type hypersensitivity, graft versus host, and allograft rejection reactions. These cells proliferate subsequent to stimulation with allogenic and foreign antigens and can liberate various mediators.

A. Effects of Anti-Id Antibodies on the Proliferative Response

Alloantigens as well as foreign antigens can induce the proliferation of T cells measured by the incorporation of [^{3}H]thymidine. While the proliferative response of T cells induced by alloantigens can be obtained with lymphocytes from normal animals, the proliferative response induced by foreign antigens can be obtained only with lymphocytes from sensitized animals. Thus, the proliferation of lymphocytes in MLC can be considered as *in vitro* primary response, whereas the proliferation induced by foreign antigens can be considered as *in vitro* secondary response, an equivalent of a delayed-type hypersensitivity reaction.

There are several lines of evidence which indicate that the T cells which proliferate following stimulation with alloantigens or foreign antigens express Id markers.

1. Responding T Cells to Foreign Antigens

The demonstration that Id determinants are expressed on the immune T cells which proliferate subsequent to stimulation with foreign antigens came from the inhibition experiments with anti-Id antibodies.

Geczy *et al.* (1976) studied the proliferation of guinea pig immune T cells induced by penicilloylated bovine γ-globulin (PO-BGG). Anti-PO-BGG antibodies were used to prepare syngeneic and homologous anti-Id antibodies (e.g., syngeneic antibodies have been obtained by injection of strain 2 anti-PO-BGG antibodies into strain 2, and homologous anti-Id antibodies by injection of antibodies produced by strain 2 into strain 13). These anti-Id antibodies were used to study the inhibition of blast response of immune T cells from strains 2, 13, and (2×13) F$_1$. The specificity of inhibition of the proliferative response was studied on the immune T cells originating from animals immunized with unrelated antigens [i.e., (T-G)-A--L and aspiryl ovalbumin) or on the proliferation induced by lectins, such as PHA.

Several interesting observations arose from this study. First, the inhibition caused by anti-Id antibodies was specific since the proliferative response to unrelated antigen as well as to lectins was not affected. This inhibition was very strong (> 90%) as assessed by the incorporation of [³H]thymidine. Second, only the syngeneic anti-Id antibodies have been inhibitory; this observation is consistent with basic ideas of the network according to the autologous anti-Id antibodies play an important role in the regulation of immune response. Third, the magnitude of the inhibition was equal in parental and F_1 T cells, indicating that allelic exclusion does not exist at T cell level. Similar suggestive results were reported by Krammer et al. (1978).

It should be mentioned that no other similar results indicating that anti-Id antibodies can suppress the antigen-specific-induced blast response have been reported. In collaboration with Ronald Schwartz we have studied the effects of BAB14 anti-Id antibodies against BALB/c anti-OVA antibodies on the OVA-induced specific proliferation of BALB/c immune T cells. We did not find any significant alteration of the proliferative response of peritoneal or lymph node T cells caused by anti-Id antibodies. In collaboration with Samuel Broder we prepared in guinea pigs three anti-Id antibodies specific for chromatography affinity-purified anti-tetanus toxoid, anti-diphtheria toxoid, and anti-KLH antibodies from the same human subject. These anti-Id antibodies inhibited the polyclonal PFC response against tetanus toxoid, diphtheria toxoid, and KLH but have no effect on the antigen-specific response of T cells.

Therefore, excepting the clear-cut results obtained in guinea pigs, no other observations have been reported concerning that Id determinants are expressed on the surface of T cells which proliferate after the stimulation by antigens.

2. MLC-Responding T Cells

Two separate lines of evidence strongly suggest that T cells which proliferate in the MLC express Id determinants on their receptors. First, the pretreatment of the T cells with anti-Id antisera and C ablated the proliferative response to alloantigens. Second, it was shown that anti-Id antibodies can induce proliferation of T cells in lieu of alloantigens.

Binz et al. (1974) have shown that the treatment of Lewis cells with anti-Id antiserum (Lewis anti-DA) and C ablated the response induced by DA cells. Similarly an anti-(Lewis anti-BN) antibody specifically inhibited Lewis anti-BN MLC response. The third party response (e.g., Lewis anti-August) was not significantly affected by these anti-Id antisera.

Similar experiments performed in mice have permitted a fine analysis of Id determinants on the receptor of T cells which proliferate in MLC. It is known that the cells which proliferate in MLC belong to Lyt 1.2 phenotype, whereas the cytolytic T cells to Lyt 2^+3^+ phenotype. Binz *et al.* (1974) have found that a syngeneic C57BL/6 mice anti-(C57BL/6 anti-CBA) T blasts antiserum inhibited both MLC and the generation of cytolytic T cells (i.e., C57BL/6 anti-CBA). However, after the adsorbtion of this anti-Id serum on positively selected Lyt 1.2 T cells, the inhibitory anti-MLC activity was removed, whereas the anti-cytolytic T cell activity remained unaltered. These results suggested that Id determinants of T cells which proliferate in MLC are different from those borne by cytolytic T cells.

The presence of Id determinants on the T cells which proliferate in MLC was considerably supported by the experiments which showed that T cells proliferate after incubation with anti-Id antibodies. Binz *et al.* (1979c) studied the kinetics and the magnitude of [^{3}H]thymidine incorporation of C57BL/6 lymphocytes stimulated with CBA cells and anti-Id antibodies against (C57BL/6 anti-CBA) T blasts. CBA-stimulating cells caused a proliferation which reached the peak at 120 hours, whereas anti-Id antibodies at 144 hours. The magnitude of [^{3}H]thymidine response at the peak of response was quite similar for both stimuli. However, in this experiment it was not shown that the same cell was stimulated by alloantigen-bearing cells and anti-Id antibodies. Only BUdR-light exposure type of experiments can clarify this point. These two groups of findings, which demonstrated that anti-Id antibodies can in the presence of C eliminate the proliferation to alloantigen in MLC or to replace the requirement for the relevant allo-MHC antigens, suggest that Id determinants are expressed on the T cells responsible for proliferative MLC response.

B. Effects of Anti-Id Antibodies on Delayed-Type Hypersensitivity Reaction

Delayed-type hypersensitivity (DTH) reaction is a cellular immune response mediated by T cells. Thus, DTH reaction can be passively transferred with sensitized lymphocytes, and the capacity of such cells to transfer DTH reaction is ablated in mice by pretreatment with anti-Thy-1.2 serum and C. It appears that the self-structures mapping to the *Ir* region are recognized in association with foreign antigens by the T cells which mediate DTH. The DTH-reactive T cells express

Lyt 1^+ antigens. Several findings suggest that DTH-reactive T cells express Id determinants.

The presence of Id determinants on the receptor of effector T cells of DTH reaction was first reported by Julius *et al.* (1977) which showed that the injection of low doses of anti-T15IdX antibodies prepared BALB/c mice for DTH response provoked by injection of R36A pneumococcal vaccine into the ears of mice. These results indicated that the DTH-reactive T cells which bear PC-binding receptors have been stimulated by anti-Id5IdX antibodies, since these receptors carried T15Id. Therefore, the antigen-binding receptor of PC-DTH-reactive T cells appeared to be similar to the binding site of TEPC15 myeloma protein. Yamamoto *et al.* (1979) explored the presence of Id determinants on DTH-reactive T cells in an experimental system in which the DTH reaction was induced by injection into the footpads of PC-coupled to peritoneal cells (PEC) followed 5 days later by challenge with PC-SC. This reaction was specific since the challenge with TNP-SC failed to cause DTH reaction. The immune T cells were able to transfer the PC-DTH reaction in normal animals, and this property was ablated by anti-Thy-1.2 + C pretreatment of the cells.

The administration of anti-T15Id antibodies (i.e., A/J anti-T15 serum) immediately before or just after preparatory injection significantly decreased the PC-specific DTH response. Administration of anti-Id antibodies before or after the challenge with PC-SC failed to alter the DTH response.

The results suggest that the PC-binding receptor of DTH-reactive T cells bears T15Id. The immunoreactivity of these cells is regulated by suppressor T cells. The administration of anti-T15Id antibodies into normal BALB/c mice generated suppressor T cells which were active in both inductor and effector phases of DTH reaction. Indeed, when BALB/c mice sensitized at day 0 with PC-PEC have been injected at day 0 or day 5 with T cells from animals pretreated with anti-T15Id antibodies, the DTH reaction caused by injection of PC-SC at day 5 was significantly altered.

Both groups of results which showed that anti-Id antibodies can replace the antigen-sensitizing injection or can block the sensitization of the PC-DTH-reactive T cells by PC-PEC demonstrated that PC-specific DTH-reactive T cells express the T15Id determinants.

Similar results have been obtained by Sy *et al.* (1980) in the azoben-zoarsonate (ABA) antigenic system. These authors succeeded in priming the ABA-specific DTH-reactive T cells by administration of rabbit anti-Id antibodies following three different experimental protocols: (a) subcutaneous injection of anti-Id antibodies, (b) intravenous injection of F(ab')$_2$ fragments, and (c) intravenous injection of anti-Id antibodies in animals pretreated with cyclophosphamide. This precaution was necessary since intravenous administration of anti-Id antibodies generates suppressor T cells (Nisonoff *et al.*, 1977).

In these experiments the mice sensitized with anti-Id antibodies have been challenged 5 days later with *p*-arsanilic acid. This reaction can be transferred in naive recipients by lymph node lymphocytes from animals pretreated with anti-Id antibodies. In ABA as in PC system, Sy *et al.* (1980) have shown that ABA-specific DTH-reactive Id$^+$ T cells are subject to regulatory effects exerted by Id-specific suppressor T cells.

The appearance of Id$^+$ ABA-specific DTH-reactive T cells, as well as of Id-specific T cells, is linked to heavy chain *Igh-1^e* allotype. Indeed, anti-IdX ABA antibodies were active only in C.AL20 and A/J mice but not in BALB/c mice.

These expected results confirmed those reported by other authors which showed that the expression of Id determinants on the receptor of T cells reactive to alloantigens, of helper T cells, and of idiotype-specific suppressor T cells is linked to *Igh-C* haplotype.

We interpreted the linkage of Id determinants of the receptor of helper and suppressor T cells to a particular *Ig-1* haplotype not as a direct control by *Igh-C* genes of *V* genes expressed by T cells.

The development of these effector, helper, or suppressor T cells may be indirectly controlled by *Ig* genes in that such cells may expand as a result of exposure to Id-bearing B cells, the presence of which appears to be determined by *IgC-h* genes. This explanation appears likely particularly in the case in which T cells are specific for idiotypes (Bona and Paul, 1979b).

One of the important observations of this study was the demonstration of a possibility to prime ABA-specific DTH-reactive T cells with F(ab')$_2$ fragments of rabbit anti-Id antibodies. Pawlak *et al.* (1973b) have shown that incomplete anti-Id antibody molecules failed to induce suppression. This indicates that the activation of suppressor T cells requires Fc fragment necessary for a cross-linking of antigen-specific receptor of T cells to Fc receptors, whereas the activiation of DTH-reactive T cells can be achieved by interaction solely between antigen-binding receptor and anti-Id antibody molecule.

In sum, in both PC and ABA antigenic systems it was shown that anti-Id antibodies can activate the DTH-reactive T cells since they express the corresponding Id determinants and suppressor T cells. These suppressor T cells have as target not only Id-bearing B cells but also the Id-bearing DTH-reactive T cells.

Therefore, these findings indicate that in certain situations the interaction between T and B cells or T and T cells are idiotype restricted and governed by the products of V region genes.

A highly relevant observation accounting for the functional immune network mechanism of regulation of immune response was provided by Sy *et al.* (1979c), who studied the contact sensitivity reaction of mice to 2,4-dinitrofluorobenzene (DNFB). The contact sensitivity reaction to DNFB is a transient phenomenon which occurs on day 5 and declines by day 9. This DNFB sensitivity can be transferred by lymph node lymphocytes in naive mice. Interestingly, the 9–15 day serum from mice which developed a DTH reaction by day 5 was able to ablate the ability of immune lymph node lymphocytes to transfer the contact-sensitivity reaction. The inhibitory factor of these sera behaves as an anti-idiotype autoantibody, since it was removed by anti-mouse Ig immunoadsorbant and immune lymph node cells. By contrast, its inhibitory activity was not altered by DNP-KLH or anti-DNP antibody immunoadsorbant. Therefore, the anti-Id antibodies which occur spontaneously during a DTH reaction can be responsible for the decline of cell-mediated immune response. These results can explain the presence of suppressor B cells which exert their effects on DTH-reactive T cells (Katz *et al.*, 1974) or on T cells which proliferate subsequent to specific antigenic stimulation (Bona *et al.*, 1976; Eyquem and Bona, 1977). In fact, these suppressor B cells which exert their effects on various subsets of T lymphocytes could secrete anti-Id antibodies which alter the function of these cells.

C. Effector Cells of Graft versus Host Reaction

Graft versus host (GVH) reaction is mediated by a subset of T cells which bears a receptor specific for alloantigen and expresses the Id determinants of anti-alloantigen antibodies. A specific GVH resistance can be obtained by injection of small concentrations of parenteral cells in F_1 hybrids. Indeed these F_1 hybrids become resistant to local or systemic GVH reaction. The GVH resistance is also mediated by T cells (Belgrau and Wilson, 1978).

Binz and Wizgell (1975c) demonstrated the presence of Id determinants on the receptor of cells which mediate GVH reaction in rats.

The allo-reactive T cells from Lewis rats were purified on beads coated with anti-Id antibodies. Anti-Id antibodies have been prepared in $(L \times DA)$ F_1 hybrids injected with Lewis T cells.

In Binz's experiments the T cells were obtained by elimination of the B cells on anti-rat Ig antibody–bead columns. Then the T cells were incubated with anti-Id antibodies and passed over the anti-rat Ig columns. The T cells which were covered by anti-Id antibodies were recovered from these columns by mechanical procedure.

The cells enriched by anti-Id (Lewis anti-DA) antibodies caused GVH reaction in $(L \times DA)$ F_1 rats but not in $(L \times BN)$ or $(L \times AN)$ F_1 hybrids. Similarly, the T cells enriched by anti-Id (Lewis anti-BN) antibodies caused GVH reaction in $(L \times BN)$ F_1 but not in $(L \times DA)$ F_1 or $(L \times AN)$ F_1 hybrids. A striking, positive correlation was observed between the percentage of anti-DA-specific Id^+ T cells and GVH reacitivity against DA. These results suggested that Id^+ T cells specific for DA alloantigen do comprise the effector T cells of GVH reaction.

Braun and Saal (1977) demonstrated that mouse GVH-reactive T cells shared Id determinants with anti-alloantigen antibodies. This was demonstrated by the ability of anti-Id antisera and C pretreatment to eliminate the GVH-reactive T cells.

Anti-Id antibodies have been prepared by injection of BALB/c anti-AKR serum in (BALB/c $\times$ AKR)F_1 hybrids. The treatment of BALB/c cells with anti-Id serum + C ablated their ability to cause a GVH reaction in F_1 mice.

These two independent studies performed in mice and rats indicated that the receptor of GVH-reactive T cells expressed the phenotypic markers of V region.

The elegant studies of Belgrau and Wilson (1979) indicated that T cells which mediated the resistance to GVH reaction bear receptors specific for MHC-encoded antigens of the GVH-reactive T cells. These receptors expressed Id determinants which are of a limited polymorphism. They showed that $(A \times B)F_1$ rats immunized against T cells from an A donor are resistant against GVH reaction induced by T cells from donor A as well as from $(A \times C)$, $(A \times D)$ . . . $(A \times N)F_1$ T cells.

Therefore, the fact that GVH reaction extended to cells of a series of other MHC types reacting against B antigens suggests that the receptor of A,C,D, . . . , N strains of rats share the Id determinants. These surprising results indicated that MHC antigen-specific receptors of T cells responsible for resistance to GVH are idiotypically similar. Wilson *et al.* (1979) proposed two explanations for this limited polymorphism of Id determinants of receptor of T cells: (a) the receptor specific for alloantigens of T cells of two strains are polymorphic gene products but are similar because they are encoded in the shared haplotype of MHC; (b) that these receptors are gene products of a conservative nonpolymorphic locus encoded by a germ-line gene which is located in chromosomes other than MHC locus.

D. Cytotoxic T Cells

Cytotoxic T cells represent another subset of effector T cells which mediates the immune specific lysis of target cells. In mice this subset expresses the Lyt 2^+3^+ antigens and does not bear the Ia antigens. The cytotoxic T cells recognize MHC (K and D in mice)-associated antigens.

With regard to the expression of Id determinants on the receptor of cytolytic T cells, the reported results show that cytolytic T cells specific for alloantigens carry the phenotypic markers of V region genes, whereas cytolytic T cells for the antigen-modified self cells do not.

Binz *et al.* (1979a) have shown that incubation of normal T cells with anti-Id antibodies can induce H-2-specific killer cells. The anti-Id antibodies used in these experiments have been prepared in C57BL/6 mice by immunization with C57BL/6 anti-CBA T blasts. Normal C57BL/6 mice T lymphocytes were incubated with 0.1–0.3% anti-Id serum, and their ability to lyse $H-2^k$, $H-2^b$ Cr-labeled target cells were then tested. In these experiments it was observed that the CBA/spleen cells as well as anti-Id antibodies induced specific killer T lymphocytes capable of lysing CBA but not BALB/c targets. Similar results have been obtained when a purified Lyt $1^-2^+3^+$ T cell population was stimulated by anti-Id antibodies. These results indicate that the receptor of cytolytic T cells specific for MHC antigens expressed Id determinants which have been the sites of stimulating properties of anti-Id antibodies.

By contrast, Sherman *et al.* (1978) and Hurme *et al.* (1980) failed to demonstrate the presence of Id determinants on cytolytic T cells specific for p-azophenylarsonate and NP-compled syngeneic cells, respectively.

In these experiments the cytolytic T cells have been induced by immunization with syngeneic cells coupled with antigen. The pretreatment of cytolytic T cells with anti-Id antibodies + C did not alter significantly their cytolytic activity.

However, a considerable body of evidence has demonstrated that the effector T cells which proliferate specifically subsequent to stimulation with allo- or foreign antigens, which mediate GVH and DTH reactions as well as cytolytic T cells specific for H-2 antigens, express the phenotypic markers of V region genes. Furthermore, the Id determinants borne on the receptor of these effector T cell subsets serve as sites of regulation of functions of these cells. Indeed, anti-Id antibodies can either suppress the function of these cells in various cell-mediated immune responses or in certain conditions can replace the antigen by stimulating the function of these cells.

IV. Idiotypic Determinants on Helper T Cells

The helper T cells (T_h) represent a subset of T lymphocyte population which cooperates with B cells to maturate and secrete antibodies in response to T-dependent antigens. The helper function of this subset is mediated by products liberated by T_h cells known as helper T factors. The antigens associated with the membrane of T_h cells are encoded by genes located in various chromosomes. Thus, Thy antigens are encoded by genes located on chromosome 9, the Lyt 1 on chromosome 19. T_h cells do not carry Ia antigens. The T_h cells recognize the antigenic determinants in association with different regions of their own MHC locus, particularly with Ir region antigenic determinants.

Therefore, the interaction between T_h and B cells is restricted by Ir genes. In Mitchinson's model (1971) the collaboration between T_h and B cells is ensured by an antigenic bridge in which the T_h cells recognize the carrier, whereas the B cells the haptens. According to this model there is no clonal restriction of the T_h and B interaction since the T cells specific for carrier can stimulate a large number of B clones specific for various haptens coupled to the same carrier. However, during the last years, several findings suggested that B cells are the subject of various subsets of T_h cells and particularly of T_h cells specific for antigenic determinants of Ig molecules. In fact, it was shown that there are T_h cells specific for isotypic, allotypic, and idiotypic determinants of Ig molecules and that the interaction between these T_h and B cells is restricted. Paricularly the interaction between Id^+-bearing T_h and B cells is clonally restricted, since these T_h cells can speak only with B cells sharing the same idiotypes, using a dictionary restricted to the idiotypic language. These new observations suggested the existence of two major subsets of T_h cells which exert synergistically their effects on B cells. T_{h1} cells are specific for antigen, and they require an antigenic bridge to activate B cells. T_{h2} appears to be specific for autologous antigenic determinants of Ig receptor of B cells. Janneway *et al.* (1977) considered that T_{h2} subset also carry antigen-specific receptors that are critical for their functioning.

A. Idiotypic Determinants on the Antigen-Binding Receptor of T Cells (T_{h1})

The pioneering work of Eichmann (1974) demonstrating that T_{h1} cells can be activated with guinea pig IgG_1 anti-Id antibodies indicated that the antigen-binding receptor of these cells expresses the phenotypic markers of V region genes. This observation was largely confirmed in various antigenic systems. Eichmann and Rajewsky (1975) have shown that IgG_1 fraction of anti-Id antibodies raised in guinea pig against A5AId of A/J anti-*Streptococcus* A antibodies can prime the T_{h1} as well as B cells. Two important conclusions have been drawn from this observation: (1) that antigen-binding receptor of T_1 and B cells shares the A5AId of anti-*Streptococcus* A antibodies, and (2) that anti-A5AId antibodies mimic the A-CHO (i.e., *Streptococcus* A) antigen with regard to its capacity to stimulate the T_{h1} and B cells.

In further studies Eichmann (1978) has shown that the ability of IgG_1 anti-Id antibodies to stimulate the T_{h1} cells represents a general phenomenon in this antigenic system. Indeed, IgG_1 guinea pig anti-Id antibodies against A5AId of A/J anti-A-CHO antibodies, against S117Id of BALB/c anti A-CHO antibodies, and against AKR anti-A-CHO antibodies primed efficiently A/J, BALB/c, and AKR, respectively, B as well as T_h cells. Black *et al.* (1976) have shown that the priming with anti-Id antibodies was at least as effective as priming with *Streptococcus* A antigen. The T cell origin of helper activity was demonstrated by the ability of anti-Thy 1.2 serum + C pretreatment to ablate the activity of T_h cells. The activity of these T_h cells was studied *in vitro* with B cells from animals primed with TNP. The cultures have been stimulated with *Streptococcus* A-TNP and the anti-TNP PFC response assessed for A-CHO-specific T_h cells. Black *et al.* (1976) have shown that T cells activated by anti-A5AId antibodies also activated the anti-A-CHO antibody-secreting cells. In these experiments an important difference was observed between A5AId$^+$ anti-A-CHO PFC when T_h cells originated from mice primed with *Streptococcus* A or with anti-A5AId antibodies. While only about 30% of anti-A-CHO antibody-secreting cells expressed A5AId when T cells originated from *Streptococcus* A primed animals, the majority expressed A5AId when T cells from anti-A5AId pretreated donors have been used. It thus appeared that the immunization with anti-A5AId antibodies expended selectively the cells bearing A5AId$^+$ receptor.

The requirement of T_h cells in the anti-phosphocholine (PC) response was demonstrated by Trenkner and Riblet (1975). Later, Cosenza *et al.* (1977) provided clear evidence that the PC-binding receptor of T_{h1} cells share IdX determinants of TEPC15 myeloma protein. This was shown in lethally irradiated BALB/c mice reconstituted with BSA-primed B cells and PC5-M315-primed T cells. These mice have been immunized with PC-BSA and the anti-BSA PFC response assessed for T_{h1} activity, since PC-primed T_{h1} cells interacted with BSA-primed B cells via PC-BSA bridge. The presence of T15IdX on the receptor of these PC-speific T_{h1} cells was demonstrated by the ability of anti-T15IdX antiserum administered into the recipients to ablate the T_{h1} activity. The endogenous origin of T15$^+$-PC-binding receptor of T_{h1} was demonstrated in two independent experiments. Julius *et al.* (1978b) devised an experimental protocol in which the stimulation of PC-specific T_{h1} cells by anti-T15Id antibodies was dissociated to the production of T15IdX$^+$ anti-PC antibodies. Thus, T_{h1} cells from conventional BALB/c mice (T15$^+$) or neonatally suppressed (T15$^-$) mice were used to reconstitute neonatally suppressed (T15$^-$) or normal (T15$^+$) nude BALB/c mice.

T_{h1} from T15$^-$ donor transferred into a T15$^+$ recipient could not be primed by anti-T15Id antibodies despite the existence of T15$^+$ anti-PC antibody. Conversely, T cells from T15$^+$ donors have been primed in T15$^-$ recipients and the T_{h1} cells which resulted have been specific for PC. In addition, their activity was inhibitable by anti-T15IdX antibodies. A more direct evidence was provided by Kaplan and Quintanas (1979b), who circumvented the difficulties of transfer experiments by inducing PC-T_{h1} cells by anti-T15Id antibodies in F_1 males bearing xid genetic defect. These mice are unable to make a T15$^+$

anti-PC antibody and, therefore, the T15Id$^+$-PC binding receptor of T_{h1} cells cannot be passively acquired from the "milieu intern" of the donor of T cells.

The presence of Id determinants on the T_{h1} cells was also studied in the anti-trimethylammonium (TMA) response in A/J mice. Alevy and Bellone (1979) have prepared guinea pig anti-Id antiserum against A/J anti-TMA antibodies. These antibodies have been able to prime the TMA-specific T_{h1} cells. These data indicated that TMA-specific helper T cells shared the Id determinants of anti-TMA antibodies.

These data taken collectively suggest that antigen-binding receptors of T_{h1} cells could in certain situations share Id determinants of Ig receptor of B cells. However, not all T_{h1} cells share Id determinants of B cells. In an elegant experiment Bottomly et al. (1978) have shown that the activation of PC-antibody-secreting cells induced by PC-KLH and T-dependent antigen is achieved by at least two subsets of T_h cells. These authors have also taken the advantage of xid defect of (CBA/N × BALB/c)F_1 males with regard to the T15$^+$ anti-PC response to study the specificity of T_h cells. The activity of KLH-T_h cells of F_1 males (T15$^-$) and F_1 females (T15$^+$) was tested with regard to their ability to interact with B cells from PC-primed F_1 females. T cells from both F_1 males or females interacted with PC-primed B cells (i.e., of F_1 females) to develop a vigorous anti-PC response to PC-KLH.

While the T cells from F_1 females have been able to mount a T15$^+$-anti-PC response, the T cells from F_1 males failed to help the expression of T15$^+$ component of anti-PC response.

These findings are in agreement with the early observations by Black et al. (1976) which indicated that the anti-A-CHO antibody-secreting cells are the subject of the help of two kinds of T_h cells, one which is primed by Streptococcus A and is able to activate A5AId$^+$ and A5AId$^-$ anti-A-CHO antibody-secreting cells, and another primed with anti-A5AId antibody which activated preferentially the A5AId$^+$ anti-A-CHO antibody-secreting cells.

The preferential interaction between Id$^+$ T_{h1} with Id$^+$ B cells is supported by several observations. Ward et al. (1978a) have shown that the transfer of T cells from donors immunized with KLH and of B cells from donors immunized with BGG-Ars in recipients immunized then with KLH-Ars produced 41 μg/ml anti-Ars antibodies from which 20 μg/ml expressed IdX. However, when positively selected Lyt 1$^+$ T_{h1} cells were pretreated with anti-Id antibodies, the amount of Id$^+$ anti-Ars antibodies was drastically decreased despite the ability of the recipient mice to make anti-Ars antibodies. From these data it clearly appeared that KLH-specific T_{h1} cells preinjected with anti-Id antibodies were unable to provide help to Id^+ anti-arsonate B cells but interacted well with IdX^- arsonate-specific B cells. Hetzelberger and Eichmann (1978b) have also demonstrated the preferential collaboration between Id^+ helper T cells and Id^+ B cells. In these experiments B cells from mice primed with IgG_1 guinea pig anti-A5AId antibodies developed a homogeneous $A5AId^+$ anti-A-CHO antibody response independently of source of T_{h1} cells (namely, either from mice immunized with *Streptococcus* A or with anti-A5AId antibodies). By contrast, B cells from mice immunized with *Streptococcus* A developed an $A5AId^+$ anti-A-CHO response only with T_{h1} cells originating from mice primed with anti-A5AId antibodies. Furthermore, the T_{h1} cells from A5AId-suppressed mice were unable to mount an $A5AId^+$ anti-A-CHO PFC response with B cells from mice primed with anti-A5AId antibodies.

Eichmann *et al.* (1978) provided decisive evidence in favor of a direct interaction between T_{h1} and B cells sharing A5AId. In this elegant experiment he demonstrated the appearance of $A5AId^+$ anti-A-CHO PFC in absence of antigenic stimulation by incubation of T and B cells from A/J mice immunized *in vivo* with *Streptococcus* A together with small amounts of anti-A5AId antibodies. It appears that in this experiment the carrier-hapten, antigenic bridge required for the interaction between T_{h1} and B cells in the Mitchisonian model was replaced by anti-Id antibodies which bound to Id determinants of T_{h1} and B cells.

B. Idiotype-Specific Helper T Cells (T_{h2})

Janneway and Paul (1973) in an elegant experiment have demonstrated that T cells recognize the Id determinants of myeloma proteins and that the receptor of these cells have anti-Id activity. Cosenza *et al.* (1977) provided clear evidence supporting the existence of Id-specific T_{h2} cells. Lethally irradiated BALB/c mice have been reconstituted with B cells from donors primed with DNP-KLH and T cells from donors primed with TEPC15. Then these mice have been immunized with DNP_6-T15 and the anti-TNP PFC response assessed for the activity of T_{h2} cells. This response was 15-fold higher than the background, indicating that T15IdX-specific T cells have been induced in the BALB/c donors immunized with TEPC15. The recipients immunized with DNP_6-MOPC630 conjugate did not develop a significant anti-DNP response. These data, as well as those of Janneway and Paul (1973), indicated that T_h cells have the ability to discriminate between Id determinants of TEPC15 and MOPC630-PC-binding myeloma proteins.

Adorni *et al.* (1979) studied the Id specificity of T_h cells in the anti-hen lysozyme antibody response. They found that two distinct subsets of T_h cells participate to this response. One type, T_{h1}, can be removed by plates coated with antigen (i.e., hen lysozyme), and another, T_{h2}, can be removed with idiotype (i.e., anti-hen lysozyme antibodies)-coated plates. Interestingly, these two subsets synergized in the anti-hen lysozyme response. Therefore, it appears that in order to obtain a maximal T–B interaction, these two subsets T_{h1} and T_{h2} should be present. Whether these two T_h cells interact with the same B cell or deliver independent signals remains to be elucidated.

Eichmann *et al.* (1978) have shown that idiotype-specific T_{h2} cells are able to deliver a maturational signal for B cells to express their program even in the absence of antigen. They observed that incubation of spleen cells (B cells) from mice primed with IgG_1 anti-A5AId antibodies together with spleen cells (T cells) from mice immunized with A5A protein led to the appearance of anti-A-CHO PFC in the absence of antigen. Therefore, the interaction between helper T cells with anti-A5AId activity with A5AId$^+$-bearing B cells was solely able to activate B cells. We have also observed a significant increase of E109IdX$^+$ anti-inulin (Inu) PFC in the absence of antigen by incubation of B cells from BALB/c mice immunized with Inu-BA and T cells from CB20 immunized with E109 myeloma protein. Similar results have been obtained using B cells from A/J mice immunized with Inu-BA and T cells from A/J mice immunized with E109 myeloma protein (Bona, 1979a).

This antigen-independent increase of anti-inulin response was highly specific, since (a) T cells from CB20 immunized with XRPC24 galactan-binding myeloma protein did not increase the E109IdX$^+$ anti-Inu PFC response above the background; and (b) T cells from CB20 immunized with E109 myeloma protein did not stimulate the appearance of anti-Inu PFC when they have been incubated with B cells from CB20 mice. CB20 mice are H-2^d which possess *Igh-C* and *Igh-V* genes of C57BL/Ka mice and therefore are unable to develop an E109IdX$^+$ anti-Inu response (Table 5.5).

The results of these experiments indicate that Id-specific helper T

TABLE 5.5

E109 Id Specific T Helper Activity[a]

10^6 B cells from mice immunized with Inu-BA	Strain donor of 10^6 T cells	Donor of T cells immunized with	Culture incubated with			
			nil		Inu-BA	
			Total[b]	% E109+	Total	% E109
BALB/c	—	—	34 ± 6	67 ± 9	144 ± 70	38 ± 10
	C.B20	None	32 ± 13	15 ± 7	123 ± 42	51 ± 17
		E109	158 ± 50	71 ± 24	226 ± 38	82 ± 10
		XPC24	35 ± 5	35	153 ± 37	35
C.B20	—	—	2 ± 0	0	2 ± 1	0
	C.B20	None	0	0	3 ± 9	0
		E109	2 ± 1	0	1 ± 1	0
		XPC24	0	0	2 ± 0	0
A/He	—	—	36 ± 5	23 ± 18	286 ± 32	36 ± 14
	A/He	None	59 ± 20	36 ± 8	321 ± 43	16 ± 8
		E109	95 ± 24	85 ± 6	205 ± 36	78 ± 18
		MOPC460	25 ± 4	0	232 ± 40	25
		XPC24	23 ± 2	36	308 ± 37	45 ± 26
		A48	33 ± 15	0	270 ± 12	67

[a] From Bona, 1979c.

[b] Anti-Inu PFC/10^6. E109 is an inulin-binding myeloma protein, whereas XPC24 binds galactan, A48 binds grass levan, and MOPC460 binds DNP and TNP.

cells can interact directly with Id-bearing B cells and deliver a maturational signal. This kind of interaction could play a role in the physiological network ensuring low concentrations of idiotypes in the absence of antigenic stimulation.

Jorgensen *et al.* (1977) have studied the specificity of ^{315}Id-specific T_{h2} cells. They primed the T_{h2} cells with isolated light and heavy chains of MOPC315 and they observed that the light chain was more efficient to induce T_{h2} cells.

In further studies Jorgensen and Hannestad (1979) have shown that V_H fragment, in contrast to V_L fragment of MOPC135, did not induce detectable helper T cell activity. In this regard even the Fv fragment of MOPC315 was inferior to V_L fragment. It is possible that preferential ability of T_{h2} cells to recognize the antigenic determinants of V region of light chain can be a general phenomenon.

C. Idiotypic Determinants on Helper T Factor

The interaction between T_h cells and B cells is mediated by soluble factors. A variety of such factors able to activate B cells has been identified in the fluid of T cell cultures (Schimpl and Wecker, 1972; Feldman, 1972; Hunter and Kettman, 1974). The helper factors can be divided into two categories: (a) nonspecific helper factors which behave like polyclonal B cell mitogens and which could exert their activity across allogenic barrier and are not clonally restricted (Amerding and Katz, 1975) and (b) antigen-specific factors which exert their activity only on syngeneic or autologous B cells and which are clonally restricted (Munro *et al.,* 1974).

Because the Id determinants are V region markers of a clone or few related clones specific for a particular antigen, theoretically, only the specific helper factors could bear Id determinants. The Id determinants have been identified on a human tetanus toxoid-specific helper T factor. Geha *et al.* (1977) showed that *in vitro* stimulation of human T lymphocytes with tetanus toxoid leads to the liberation of a helper factor able to stimulate autologous B cells to produce antitetanus toxoid antibodies. Anti-Id antibodies have been prepared in rabbits against anti-tetanus toxoid antibodies isolated from healthy human subjects. Mudawwar *et al.* (1978) used these anti-Id antibodies to identify the Id determinants on tetanus toxoid-specific helper T factor. The helper activity was removed by passage over anti-Id antibody immunoadsorbants and was not altered after the passage over anti-human IgG or IgM antibody immunoadsorbants.

Mozes and Haimovich (1979) have also shown that a murine antigen-specific T cell factor shares IdX with antibodies of the same specificity. The presence of IdX of anti (T,G)-AL antibodies linked to $Ig-1^b$ haplotype on the (T,G)-A--L specific helper factor was investigated. The specificity of the helper factor was demonstrated by the ability of antigen–Sepharose columns to adsorb the helper activity produced by educated T cells from C3H.SW, CWB, and C3H/DiSm strains of mice. The activity of the factor was completely removed by passage over anti-Id antibody immunoadsorbant.

These observations indicated that helper factor and antigen-binding receptor of T cells share Id determinants of humoral antibodies. In summary, it therefore appears that B cells are the subject of effects of various subsets of helper T cells.

One subset, T_{h1}, which is not clonally restricted, interacts with B cells via a carrier–hapten bridge. Some of T_{h1} which expresses Id determinants on their receptor interacts preferentially with Id^+-bearing B cells through an anti-Id antibody bridge can lead to the maturation of B cells in the absence of antigens.

The second subset specific for idiotypes (i.e., anti-idiotypic), T_{h2} cells, can be stimulated by the products of B cells, i.e., by Id-bearing antibodies. Probably, these anti-Id T_{h2} cells share Id determinants of anti-Id antibodies. No available data exist with this regard. At first glance these cells are able to interact directly with and activate the B cells by an idiotype–anti-idiotype complementary reaction. This kind of interaction observed only *in vitro* can represent a simply artificial situation. However, it can play an important role in the immune network by ensuring low concentrations of idiotypes in the absence of antigenic stimulation. The important regulatory role of this second subset of T_{h2} which can be specific for isotypic, allotypic, or idiotypic antigenic determinants of Ig receptor of B cells can provide a fine tuning of the regulation of expression of class, allotype, and idiotype of antibodies during the immune response.

V. Idiotypic Determinants on Suppressor T Cells

The suppressor T cells represent another subset of T lymphocyte population which plays an important role in the regulation of humoral and cell-mediated immune responses. Suppressor T cells (T_s) have a receptor specific for antigens but lack membrane-associated structures which recognize self-specificities. Therefore, their effects are not

MHC restricted. For the murine system, T_s cells have the phenotype Lyt $1^-2^+3^+$, and they express I-J antigens. In human systems, T_s cells have receptors for Fc γ and bear OKT_8 antigens. They exert the suppressor effects on T_h cells or directly on B cells. These suppressor properties are mediated by suppressor factors.

With regard to the idiotypic specificities of T_s, they can be divided into two categories: T_s cells specific for antigens which share Id determinants with humoral antibodies and T_s specific for idiotype (i.e., bearing receptor exhibiting anti-Id specificity).

A. Id Determinants on Antigen-Specific T_s Cells

In his pioneering work, Eichmann (1975) showed that administration of guinea pig IgG_2 anti-A5AId antibodies into A/J mice generated T_s which experted their activity on A5AId-specific T_h cells.

This observation suggested that the receptor of T_s bore A5AId determinants which were the site of stimulation of suppressor activity by anti-A5AId antibodies.

The direct evidence of the presence of Id determinants on the receptor of T_s cells was provided several years later by Lewis and Goodman (1978). These authors induced azobenzoarsonate (ABA)-specific T_s cells after injection of soluble ABA-IgG conjugate in A/J mice. The activity of these ABA-specific T_s cells was demonstrated in transfer experiments.

An anti-Id antiserum was prepared in the rabbit against A/J anti-ABA antibodies.

ABA-specific T_s cells represent 0.06% of T cell population as assessed by purification on ABA-coated plates. A majority of the cells recovered from ABA-coated plates bore the Thy-1.2 marker (95%) and exhibited the ability to bind the antigen (90%). Using staining methods Lewis and Goodman (1978) have shown that 68% of the T_s cells have been stained by anti-Ia antibodies and 54% by anti-Id antibodies. Therefore, more than half of T_s which bound ABA expressed IdX of anti-ABA antibodies. These findings represented the first demonstration that antigen-induced T_s cells, enriched on ABA-coated plates, shared Id determinants with humoral antibodies specific for the same antigen.

After this original observation, several investigators, in various antigenic systems, provided direct, functional, and indirect evidence that the antigen-specific receptor of T_s cells also expresses Id determinants.

1. Hen Lysozyme System (HEL)

Harvey *et al.* (1979) induced HEL-specific T_s cells in B10 mice, a strain which is genetically nonresponder to HEL. The activity of B10, HEL-specific T_s cells was tested *in vitro* on T_h cells induced by priming with a HEL fragment lacking an N-terminal region believed to stimulate T_s cells. A site-related anti-Id antiserum was prepared in guinea pig by immunization with B10A (a responder strain), anti-HEL antibodies. The *in vitro* pretreatment of T_s with guinea pig anti-Id antibodies and C ablated the suppressor properties of these cells. These results clearly indicated that B10, HEL-specific T_s cells share Id determinants with B10A, anti-HEL antibodies.

2. Phosphocholine (PC) System

In the PC system there are suggestive *in vivo* and *in vitro* experiments which indicate that PC-specific T_s cells express T15Id determinants, since they can be stimulated by anti-T15Id antibodies in lieu of antigen.

Bottomly *et al.* (1978), using an adoptive transfer system, have shown that the treatment of BALB/c KLH-primed T cells with rabbit anti-T15Id antibodies resulted in the occurrence of Lyt 2.2 T_s cells which specifically exert their effects on T_h cells for the secondary antibody response of PC-primed B cells to PC-KLH.

These T_s cells induced by anti-T15Id antibodies seem to be specific for T15Id as well as for carrier. Indeed, T_s cells had no effect on the anti-PC antibody response induced by PC coupled to a heterologous carrier and did not alter the anti-TNP antibody response elicited by TNP-KLH conjugate. Kim (1979) has reported that the incubation of normal BALB/c cells with anti-T15IdX antibodies together with R36A pneumococcal vaccine generated T_s cells. The activity of these T_s cells was measured in cocultures with fresh normal BALB/c spleen cells. The T cell origin of the suppressor cells was demonstrated by the ability of anti-Thy 1.2 antiserum + C pretreatment to ablate the suppressor activity. Induction of T_s cells by anti-T15IdX antibodies as in Bottomly's experiments suggests that T_s cells express T15IdX. However, they can be specific for T15IdX. No available data have been provided with regard to the Id determinants of the receptor of these T_s cells. More likely these T_s cells bear T15IdX and, therefore, can be stimulated by anti-T15IdX antibodies as in Eichmann's system, in which the anti-A5AIdX antibodies generated T_s cells.

3. Phenyltrimethylammonium (TMA) System

Alevy *et al.* (1980) have described the anti-TMA response of A/J mice, which is characterized by an IdX expressed on 50% of anti-TMA antibodies.

In further studies Alevy *et al.* (1980) developed an experimental system in which monovalent antigens tyr (TMA) generated TMA-specific T_s cells. Interestingly, the activity of these TMA-specific T_s cells is idiotype restricted, since only the PFC-secreting IdX^+ anti-TMA antibodies have been suppressed in the A/J mice injected with monovalent tyr TMA. The injection of anti-TMA IdX antibodies in lieu of antigen-generated T_s cells indicates that these cells bear similar idiotypes with anti-TMA antibodies. This study first showed that tyr TMA can activate preferentially a subset of TMA suppressor T cells which share Id determinants with humoral antibodies and that the activity of T_s cells is idiotype restricted.

4. T_sCells Specific for Delayed-Type Hypersensitivity (DTH) Reaction

Benecerraf's group provided several direct and functional evidence that T_s cells which exert their acitivity on effector T cells of DTH reaction express Id determinants on their surface. This was demonstrated in two different antigenic systems, namely, azobenzoarsonate (ABA) and 4-hydroxy-3-nitrophenyl acetyl (NP). Delayed-type hypersensitivity reaction to ABA hapten can be provoked in A/J mice by injecting subcutaneously ABA coupled with syngeneic spleen cells.

Sy *et al.* (1979a) have shown that either the injection of rabbit anti-ABA IdX antibodies or IdX^+ anti-ABA antibody coupled to syngeneic cells caused a significant reduction of ABA-specific DTH reaction. This inhibition was due to the T_s cells, since (a) the suppression was transferrable in normal recipients; (b) the activity of these cells was ablated by anti-Thy-1.2 antibody $+C$ treatment; and (c) the occurrence of suppressor cells was present by administration of low doses of cyclophosphamide.

Interestingly, the T_s cells occurred only in the strains of mice of $Ig-1^c$ haplotype. The IdX of anti-ABA antibodies is also linked to

Ig-1[c.] The preliminary data announced by the authors indicate that anti-Id antibody +C treatment of T_s cells abolishes the suppressor activity.

Weinberg and Hall (1979) have taken advantage of well-defined idiotypic NP systems developed by Mäkelä to study the presence of V-h^{NP} Id on T_s cells which exert their effects on NP-specific effector T cells of DTH reaction.

The fine specificity pattern and the genetics of NP-specific effector T cells of DTH reaction induced by injection of NP-coupled syngeneic cells were similar to the humoral anti-NP antibodies. The T_s cells have been obtained only in mice bearing *Ig-1*^{b} haplotype. The NP-Id is also linked to *Ig-1*^{b} allotype (Mäkelä *et al.,* 1977).

Interestingly, the SJL strain, which is unable to develop a heteroclitic NPId$^+$ response because they are weak λ chain makers, generated T_s cells. This observation indicated the endogenous origin of receptor of T_s cells as well as that these cells do not use L λ chain to make their receptors.

The presence of Id determinants on Ts cells was demonstrated by the ability of anti-Id antibody +C treatment to ablate the suppressor activity. Furthermore, the activity of NP-specific suppressor T cells from a CBA strain (Ig-1^j) was not altered by anti-NP^b Id antibody +C treatment.

These results indicate that antigen-specific T_s cells which exert their activity directly on the B cells as in TMA system, on T_h cells as in *Streptococcus* A, PC, HEL systems, or on effector cells of DTH reaction share Id determinants with humoral antibodies.

Direct evidence on the Id determinants associated with the membrane of these T_s cells was provided by staining and cytotoxic techniques. Functional evidence was provided by the experiments in which anti-Id antibody treatment generated T_s cells in the absence of antigen.

B. Idiotype-Specific Suppressor T Cells

In contradistinction to the antigen-specific T_s cells which should not be clonally restricted, the Id-specific T_s cells (having a receptor with anti-Id activity) should exert their effects only on the clones secreting Id$^+$-bearing antibodies. A striking parallel can be drawn between these Id-specific T_s cells and T_{h2} cells, since their effects are idiotype restricted. Naturally occurring and antibody-induced Id-specific T_s cells have been described.

The receptor of these T_s cells lack the ability to bind the antigen.

1. Naturally Occurring T_s Cells

We have shown that TNP-BL and TNP-NWSM induced primary *in vitro* anti-TNP antibody response and that 10–20% of anti-TNP-secreted antibodies expressed the 460-Id (Bona and Paul, 1979a). The 460-Id$^+$ component of anti-TNP PFC response to TNP-NWSM was substantially greater in spleen cell cultures pretreated with anti-Thy-1.2 serum and C than in unseparated spleen cells. Furthermore, the addition of nylon wool-purified T cells to the spleen B cells strongly inhibited the 460-Id$^+$ component of anti-TNP response (Table 5.6). These results suggested that the nonimmunized BALB/c mice contained a discrete population of T cells which regulate the expression of B lymphocytes able to secrete 460-Id$^+$ antibodies.

In further experiments we characterized the properties of these naturally occurring Ts cells as shown below.

a. SPECIFICITY OF NATURALLY OCCURRING T_s CELLS

The specificity of T_s cells which regulate the 460-Id$^+$ component of anti-TNP response was studied by plate-binding experiments. The suppressor activity was removed by incubation of these T cells on petri dishes coated with MOPC460. It was not altered subsequent to incubation on petri dishes coated with EPC109 and MOPC167 myeloma proteins (which bear unrealted idiotypes), with monoclonal anti-460Id antibodies, or TNP-BSA. In addition, we have shown that T cells recovered from MOPC460-coated dishes exhibited a stronger inhibitory capacity, per cell basis, than the T-enriched population (Table 5.7). These results clearly showed that regulatory T_s cells of 460-Id$^+$ component of anti-TNP response have been specific for 460Id, (Bona and Paul, 1979a). It should be mentioned that these naturally occurring 460Id-specific T_s cells have been stimulated subsequent to immunization with MOPC460 myeloma protein, which induced an anti-460Id immunity. Per cell basis, the suppressor activity was stronger in the mice immunized with MOPC460 than in normal mice (Table 5.8). These data clearly showed that 460Id-bearing molecules not only can be bound by the receptor of T_s but can expand these cells (Bona *et al.*, 1979a).

TABLE 5.6

Inhibitory Effect of T Cells on the Development of PFC-Secreting Anti-TNP Antibodies Bearing 460Id[a]

Origin of cells	Total anti-TNP PFC/culture	460-Id$^+$ PFC/culture	460-Id$^+$ PFC (%)
BALB/c spleen cells (unseparated)	147 ± 7[b]	14 ± 8	10
BALB/c B cells obtained by anti-Thy-1.2 + C treatment	92 ± 13	37 ± 17	41
BALB/c B cells + nylon wool-purified T-cells	110 ± 6	−12 ± 9	−10
BALB/c B cells + T cells treated with anti-Thy-1.2 + C	103 ± 9	27 ± 10	27
BALB/c B cells + C.B20 T cells	159 ± 12	49 ± 22	31

[a] Unseparated spleen cells or B cells were cultured in quadruplicate at 5 × 10^5 cells/microwell, with or without 5 × 10^5 T cells, with TNP-NWSM (3 μg/ml). The number of anti-TNP PFC were determined at 3 days in the absence or presence of BALB/c anti-460Id (1:100). Results reported are total anti-TNP-PFC ± SE, anti-TNP-PFC which are inhibitable by anti-460Id (460-Id$^+$ PFC) ± S.E., and percent of anti-TNP-PFC which secrete 460-Id-bearing molecules. From Bona and Paul, 1979a.

[b] Mean ± S.E. of four cultures (5 × 10^5 cells/culture).

TABLE 5.7

Idiotypic Specificity of Suppressor T Cells[a]

B cells (5 × 10⁵) cocultured with	% 460-Id⁺ PFC Exp. No.				
	1	2	3	4	5
Nothing	46[c]	52	38	55	50
5 × 10⁵ T cells	3	—[d]	11	32	19
5 × 10⁵ T cells recovered from MOPC460-coated plates	60	61	43	67	50
5 × 10⁵ T cells adsorbed on control plates[b]	4	10	0	32	0
5 × 10⁵ T cells adsorbed on control plates[b]	16	16	11	44	16
5 × 10⁵ T cells recovered from E109-coated plates	48	55	55	—	—

[a] Anti-Thy-1.2 and C-treated BALB/c spleen cells (B cells; 5 g 10⁵/well) were cultured with nothing or with 5 × 10⁵ nylon column-passed spleen cells (T cells) which had been subjected to various treatments. Total number of anti-TNP PFC and of PFC secreting 460Id-bearing molecules were measured 3 days after stimulation with TNP-NWSM (3 μg/ml). From Bona and Paul, 1979a.

[b] Control plates were as follows: experiments 1–3, E109-coated plates; experiment 4, MOPC167-coated plates; experiment 5, purified A/He anti-460Id-coated plates.

[c] Mean of percent of anti-TNP-PFC inhibitable by anti-460Id.

[d] Not done.

TABLE 5.8

Inhibitory Effect of T Cells on the Development of PFC Secreting Anti-TNP Antibodies Bearing 460ID[a]

B cells (5 × 10⁵) incubated with various number of T cells	T cells from normal BALB/c		T cells from BALB/c immunized with MOPC460	
	Anti-TNP PFC	% 460-Id⁺	Anti-TNP PFC	% 460-Id⁺
Nil	86 ± 3	69	82 ± 1	59
10⁴	157 ± 41	74	79 ± 14	19
10⁵	86 ± 24	38	66 ± 2	0
2.5 × 10⁵	96 ± 16	23	128 ± 43	3
5 × 10⁵	132 ± 10	3	110 ± 28	0

[a] B cells (5 × 10⁵) were cultured in triplicate in microtiter plates with or without various number of 460-Id-specific suppressor T cells recovered from MOPC460 coated plates and with 3 μm of TNP-NWSM. The number of anti-TNP PFC were determined at 3 days in absence or presence of BALB/c anti-460Id antibodies (1/100). From Bona et al., 1979a.

b. PHENOTYPE OF 460ID-SPECIFIC T_S CELLS

The expression of Lyt and Qa_1 antigens used in the characterization of various functional subsets of T lymphocytes was studied in another set of experiments. BALB/c-enriched T cells recovered or not from MOPC460-coated plates have been pretreated with anti-Lyt 1.2 and anti-Lyt 2.2 sera +C before to be cocultured with B cells stimulated *in vitro* with TNP-NWSM. We have observed in several experiments that anti-Lyt 2.2 serum +C treatment regularly eliminated the suppressor activity. In some, but not all, experiments, the suppressor activity was partially diminished by anti-Lyt 1.2 serum +C pretreatment.

The expression of Qa_1 antigen was studied in (C58J × BALB/c)F_1 mice, since our antiserum recognized the Qa_1 allelic form borne by C58J mice. This strain of mice has $H-2^h$ haplotype but bears the $Igh-C^a$ allotype (like BALB/c) and at least some $V-h^a$ genes. They are able to make 460-Id^+ anti-TNP antibodies.

The suppressor activity of (C58J × BALB/c)F_1 T cells (Table 5.9) was ablated by anti-Qa_1 serum +C treatment. From these data we concluded that naturally occurring 460Id-specific T_s cells, as well as those induced in BALB/c mice subsequent to immunization with MOPC460 myeloma protein, expressed Lyt 2.2 and Qa_1 antigens. However, our results cannot exclude the existence of an Lyt 1^+2^+ or Lyt 1^+2^- with suppressor activity, or an Lyt 1^+2^+ cell which helps the generation of Lyt $2^+Qa_1^+$ T cells (Bona and Paul, 1979b).

c. DETECTION OF 460ID-SPECIFIC T_S CELLS IN MICE BEARING $Ig-1^a$ ALLOTYPE

The expression of 460Id on anti-TNP antibodies appears only in the strains of mice which possess $Igh-V^a$ and $Igh-C^a$ genes of BALB/c type (Bona and Paul, 1979b; Zeldis *et al.,* 1979; Cazenave *et al.,* 1980). By contrast, several strains of mice, including the congenic strains to BALB/c, failed to express 460Id.

The study of naturally occurring 460Id-specific T_s cells have shown that only the mice having $Igh-C^a$ genes (e.g., BALB/c and C58J) also have Ts cells.

Three congenic strains of mice to BALB/c, i.e., C.AL20 Igh-C^d, C.B20 Igh-C^b, and BAB.14 Igh-V^a and Igh-C^b, failed to express a suppressor activity (Table 5.10). These results stongly suggested that the occurrence of 460Id-specific T_s cells is limited to the expression of

TABLE 5.9

Phenotype of Suppressor T Cells

5 × 10⁵ B cells incubated with	BALB/c				(C58/J × BALB/c)F₁	
	1[a]	2	3	4	1	2
—	127 ± 10[b] (40)	86 ± 2 (51)	62 ± 4 (43)	226 ± 9 (69)	30 ± 18 (44)	123 ± 16 (55)
5 × 10⁵ T cells	146 ± 14 (10)	129 ± 2 (−3)	205 ± 27 (4)	295 ± 14 (4)	142 ± 9 (5)	91 ± 7 (15)
5 × 10⁵ T Cells treated with anti-Lyt-1.2 + C	77 ± 5 (32)	35 ± 2 (27)	148 ± 24 (12)	156 ± 28 (11)	110 ± 10 (29)	99 ± 7 0
5 × 10⁵ T cells treated with anti-Lyt-2.2 + C	144 ± 22 (40)	93 ± 11 (72)	214 ± 43 (40)	240 ± 44 (54)	78 ± 12 (53)	81 ± 10 (46)
5 × 10⁵ T Cells treated with anti-TLH + C	ND[c]	ND	ND	ND	138 ± 24 (62)	105 ± 10 (38)

[a] No. of experiments.
[b] Total anti-TNP PFC ± SD; Number in parentheses = % of 460-Id⁺ anti-TNP PFC.
[c] ND, not done.

TABLE 5.10

Relationship between 460Id-Specific Suppressor T Cells and Igh-C[a] Genes

Origin of cells		460-Id⁺ anti-TNP response[a]
B cells	T cells	
BALB/c	—	+++
BALB/c	BALB/c	−
BALB/c	BAB.14	++
BALB/c	CAL.20	+++
BALB/c	C.B20	+++
C58/J	—	+++
C58/J	C58/J	−

[a] The degree of response designated in a − to +++ scale was determined from three individual experiments.

Igh-C^a allotype (Bona *et al.*, 1979b). We do not think that Igh-C^a genes directly control the specificity of the receptor (i.e., anti-Id receptor) of T_s cells. By contrast, the development of these 460Id-specific Ts cells may be indirectly controlled by Igh-C genes, since these cells may expand as result of 460-Id$^+$ antibody produced by B cells, the presence of which is under the control of Igh-C genes.

d. Site of Action of 460Id-specific T_s Cells

Results obtained in various experimental systems are consistent with the concept that T_s cells exert their suppressor activity on T_h cells. By contrast, our studies of the site of action of 460Id-specific T_s cells indicated that they exert their suppressor activity directly on B cells.

This concept is stongly supported by three sets of experiments.

1. T_s cells depleted of Lyt 1.2 cells still exhibited their inhibitory activity on B cells depleted of Lyt 1.2 cells: In this set of experiments the enriched T cells and positively selected B cells were pretreated with anti-Lyt 1.2 serum +C and then cocultured with B cells stimulated with antigen (Table 5.11). The conclusion of this experiment was that T_s cells exert their effects on B cells in the absence of Lyt 1.2 cells.

2. Failure of T cells from congenic BALB/c strains of mice to increase the suppressor activity of positively selected Lyt 2.2 BALB/c T cells: In these experiments C.B20 or C.AL20 T cells have been added to Lyt 2.2 BALB/c T cells cocultured with BALB/c B cells depleted of Lyt 1.2 cells. No increase of suppressor activity was observed, suggesting that C.B20 or C.AL20 T cells have not been able to provide a help in any direction (Table 5.12).

3. Suppression of the ability of hybridomas to lyse TNP-coated SRBC: In collaboration with D. Juy we have tested the activity of T cells from BALB/c immunized with MOPC460 on PFC response of two hybridoma-secreting IgM monoclonal antibodies; DJTNP11 is a hybridoma which secretes a 460-Id$^+$ and DJTNP12 a 460-Id$^-$ anti-TNP monoclonal antibody (Buttin *et al.*, 1979). Incubation for 72 hours of T cells with DJTNP11 hybridoma strongly inhibited the ability to make anti-TNP PFC, whereas had it no inhibitory effect on DJTNP12 hybridoma cells. These data provide evidence that Lyt 2.2, 460Id-specific T_s cells exert their suppressor activity directly on B cells.

TABLE 5.11

Effect of Suppressor T Cells Depleted of Lyt-1$^+$ Cells on 460Id Component of the Anti-TNP Response of Anti-Lyt-1.2 Serum and C Pretreated B Cells Stimulated with TNP-NWSM[a]

B cells	Treatment of B cells	T cells	Treatment of T cells	Anti-TNP PFC/culture total	% 460$^+$	Anti-TNP PFC/culture total	% 460$^+$	Anti-TNP PFC/culture total	% 460$^+$
5 × 10^5	—	—	—	86 ± 2	52	192 ± 22	25	263 ± 29	37
5 × 10^5	Anti-Lyt-1.2	—	—	41 ± 3	69	252 ± 19	24	218 ± 27	36
5 × 10^5	Anti-Lyt-2.2	—	—	97 ± 10	62	ND^b	ND	ND	ND
5 × 10^5		5 × 10^5	Anti-Lyt-1.2	79 ± 18	18	95 ± 13	0	113 ± 20	18
5 × 10^5	Anti-Lyt-1.2	5 × 10^5	Anti-Lyt-1.2	39 ± 8	30	68 ± 4	4	37 ± 8	21
5 × 10^5	Anti-Lyt-1.2	5 × 10^5	Anti-Lyt-2.2	58 ± 10	38	52 ± 10	38	41 ± 10	67

[a] The cells were cultured in microplates during 4 days in presence of 5 µg of TNP-NWSM. The anti-TNP PFC response and 460-Id$^+$ component of this response was estimated as previously.

[b] ND, not done.

TABLE 5.12

Absence of Lyt 1^+2^+ Helpers for the Induction of 460Id-Specific Suppressor T Cells

BALB/c B cells (5×10^5) pretreated with anti-Lyt 1.2 + C and incubated with		anti-TNP PFC/culture	
T cells from	BALB/c 460Id-specific T cells	Total	% 460-Id$^+$
—	—	164 ± 26	52
—	10^5	153 ± 6	14
BALB/c (10^5)	—	117 ± 11	28
BALB/c (5×10^5)	10^5	160 ± 1	18
C.B20 (5×10^5)	—	119 ± 27	60
C.B20 (5×10^5)	10^5	138 ± 15	18
C.AL20 (5×10^5)	—	153 ± 29	51
C.AL20 (5×10^5)	10^5	228 ± 58	29

Although such a cellular target of T cells would be anticipated the idiotypic specificity of T_s cells, these data provide one of the first well-documented instances of action of T_s cells directly on B cells.

2. Antibody-Induced Id-Specific Suppressor T Cells

Hart *et al.* (1972) have shown that the administration of rabbit anti-Id antibodies against A/J anti-A antibodies leads to a long-lasting suppression of IdX$^+$ anti-Ars antibody response. Owen *et al.* (1977) observed that a substantial number of T cells from A/J mice which have been idiotypically suppressed and then hyperimmunized formed rosettes with mouse RBC coated with Fab fragment of IdX$^+$ anti-Ars antibodies. A high number (8–14%) of cells exhibited the ability to form these RFC. The T cell origin of rosetting cells was demonstrated by the ability of anti-Thy 1.2 serum +C treatment to eliminate these cells. The specificity of these RFC for IdX was demonstrated in various control experiments as follows: (a) failure of cells to form rosettes with RBC coated with nonspecific Ig or IdX$^-$ anti-Ars antibody; (b) inhibition of rosettes by IdX$^+$ anti-Ars antibodies; and (c) inhibition of rosettes by F(ab′)$_2$ fragment of rabbit anti-Id antibodies but not by anti-mouse Ig antibodies; (d) inhibition of rosettes by hapten (i.e., azobenzenearsonic acid) N-acetyl-L-tyrosine and not by unrelated haptens.

The cells exhibiting the ability to rosette contained suppressor activity. Indeed the enriched T cell population depleted of Id-specific RFC T cells failed to transfer suppression, whereas the population enriched in rosetting cells was more efficient than unseparated T cells (Owen *et al.*, 1977). These Id-specific T_s cells probably interact directly with Id^+-bearing B cells.

C. *V* Region Antigenic Determinants on Suppressor Factors

The activity of T_s cells is mediated by suppressor factors. These factors can be extracted from thymocytes or T lymphocytes. They possess the capacity to bind to antigens and express I-J antigens.

The expression of *V* region antigenic markers on the suppressor factors was investigated by Tada *et al.* (1979). A "monoclonal" suppressor factor was obtained from hybridomas obtained by fusion of T_s cells with lymphoma T cell lines. The suppressor activity of these factors was removed by passage over columns coated with antigens, anti-I-J antibodies, and goat anti-mouse Fv fragment antibodies. These results indicated that the suppressor factors share nonidiotypic "framework determinants" of mouse Ig molecules. These data are in agreement with previous results which showed that V_H framework determinants are present on the receptor of T cells (Lonai *et al.*, 1978; Cazenave *et al.*, 1977b).

Idiotypic determinants have been also identified on the suppressor factors. Germain *et al.* (1979) have shown that GAT-specific suppressor factors can be removed by passage over GAT columns as well as anti-Id antibody columns. Bach *et al.* (1979) obtained similar results by studying the properties of ABA-specific suppressor T factor. These results indicate that the suppressor factor contains molecules able to bind the antigen, bearing I-J antigens and at least two categories of *V* region antigenic determinants.

In summary, the data presented in this section show that idiotypic determinants as well as framework antigenic determinants can be identified on T_s cells as well as suppressor factors. A striking parallel exists between T_s and T_h cells with regard to the Id determinants of their receptors.

Antigen-specific T_h and T_s cells as well as helper and suppressor factors share Id determinants with humoral antibodies. The activation of these cells requires antigen, but since their receptor bears Id determinants they can be activated by anti-Id antibodies in lieu of antigens.

The second category is represented by T_h and T_s cells specific for idiotype and which are activated by Id-bearing antibodies (the receptor of these cells has an anti-Id specificity). Idiotype-specific T_s cells share Id determinants with anti-Id antibodies (Bona *et al.*, 1979c).

The effects of these T cells are idiotypically restricted, and they exhibit their activity in the absence of antigen. It is not clear if the activity of these cells is mediated by factors, since no helper or suppressor factors with anti-Id activity have been identified yet. More likely the Id-specific T_h and T_s cells exert their effects directly on B cells.

VI. T Cell-Mediated Idiotype Suppression of Synthesis of Antibodies

Injection of syngeneic, homologous, or heterologous anti-Id antisera leads to a specific suppression of clones which bear the corresponding idiotype. In certain experimental systems the administration of anti-Id antibodies generates T_s cells. This type of Id suppression is mediated by T cells.

Eichmann (1974) have shown that the administration of IgG_2 subclass of guinea pigs anti-A5AId antibodies into A/J mice led to the suppression of synthesis of A5AId$^+$ anti-*Streptococcus* A antibodies. This suppression was specific since neither normal guinea pig Ig nor guinea pig anti-B72Id antibodies (B72 is a clone which bears an unrelated idiotype) have any effect on A5AId$^+$ component of anti-*Streptococcus* A antibodies. In further studies Eichmann (1975a) has shown that high concentrations of IgG_2 anti-A5AId antibodies caused an immediate but short suppression, whereas the small concentrations caused a chronic suppression which lasted for more than 1 year. Hetzelberger and Eichmann (1978a) have shown that high zone suppression was maximal 7 days after injection and declined by 21 days, whereas the low zone suppression was fully developed by 7 weeks and was tested for a long time. High dose suppression cannot be transferred, while the low dose suppression can be transferred in naive recipients. Eichmann (1975a) have shown that the suppressor capacity of cells is abolished with anti-Thy-1.2 antibody $+C$ pretreatment. In addition, the cells recovered from histamine-coated beads exhibited a stronger inhibitor activity per cell basis as compared to unseparated spleen cells. The T cells bear a receptor for histamine, and, therefore, they could be enriched on histamine columns. Hammerling and Eichmann (1976) have shown that the T_s cells express I-J alloantigens.

It is interesting to follow through the development of experimental work on idiotypic suppression of A5AId$^+$ component of anti-*Streptococcus* A antibody how the ideas on the mechanism of Id suppression had evolved.

In the early study Eichmann (1974) discovered that only IgG$_2$ subclass of anti-A5AId was able to cause suppression. Since this subclass binds to macrophages and binds complement, it was considered that the suppression is due to the elimination of cells with A5AId-bearing receptor. These cells killed by IgG$_2$ anti-A5AId antibodies +C were then eliminated through a phagocytosis process.

In 1975 new experimental data clearly indicated that the suppression is mediated by T_s cells. Eichmann (1975a) considered that these T_s cells bear a receptor which recognizes the A5AId-bearing B cells and interacted directly with these cells, since the observed idiotype suppression was clonally restricted. However, at this time he already envisaged a direct effect of T_s on another T cell subset as well. Indeed, later Eichmann *et al.* (1977) have found that the number of the precursors of A5AId-secreting B cells found in the normal or suppressed animals have not been significantly different, and therefore the concept of a direct effect of T_s on T_h cells occurred. This concept was strengthened by Hetzelberger and Eichmann (1978) findings which showed that the animal suppressed with low zone doses of anti-A5AId antibodies lack A-CHO-specific A5AId-bearing T_h cells, whereas the A5AId$^+$ precursor of B cells remain fully responder. Therefore, according to new results Eichmann considered that A5AId$^+$ T_s cells exert their effect on A5AId$^+$ T_h cells, and the inhibition of these T_h cells alters the capacity of B cells to synthesize A5AId$^+$ anti-A-CHO antibodies.

However, the attempts to kill T_s cells by IgG$_2$ anti-A5AId antibody +C were only occasionally successful (Eichmann *et al.*, 1977). Therefore, the presence of A5AId determinants on T_s cells was not yet clearly demonstrated.

The evolution of ideas on the mechanism of idiotype suppression in A5AId system represents a genuine example of dialectics of concepts and thoughts paralleled by the labor and experimental truths. The understanding of the mechanism of this idiotype suppression also led to the development of the concept of idiotype restriction of collaboration between B, T_h, and T_s during the immune response.

Hart *et al.* (1972) have also found that the administration of heterologous (i.e., rabbit) anti-Id antibodies into A/J mice led to the suppression of IdX^+ component of anti-Ars antibody response. A long-lasting suppression was obtained in the adult mice, and only 22 weeks after immunization half of the mice had recovered from suppression. This suppression cannot be obtained with $F(ab')_2$ or Fab fragments of anti-Id antibodies (Pawlak *et al.*, 1973b), indicating that the Fc fragment plays an important role in the induction of suppression.

This suppression concerns only IdX^+ components of anti-Ars antibody response since the anti-Ars antibodies bearing IdI have not been inhibited (Ju *et al.*, 1977).

Nisonoff *et al.* (1977) have shown that the suppression can be transferred in mildly irradiated recipients by spleen cells or peritoneal cells. In further elegant studies reviewed in the previous section, Owen *et al.* (1977) have shown that idiotype suppression induced by rabbit anti-IdX antibodies is mediated by idiotype-specific T_s cells which exert their effects only on IdX^+ components of anti-Ars antibodies. Ward *et al.* (1978b) have shown that the majority of these T_s cells expressed Lyt 2^+3^+ phenotype. However, Lyt 1^+2^+ cells have also been able to transfer to some extent the suppression. Whether the Lyt 1^+ cells are genuine suppressor or helper for the development of Lyt 2^+3^+ T_s cells is not yet clear.

Dohi and Nisonoff (1973) have shown that Id-specific T_s cells can also be generated by injection of IdX anti-Ars antibodies coupled to thymocytes. The induction of the Id-specific suppressor activity was not dependent of H2 type of thymocyte carriers. This new model for induction of Id-specific T_s cells sheds a light on the mechanism of generation of Id-specific T_s which can be stimulated by idiotypes, since the precursor of these T_s cells bears anti-Id receptors.

We have considered that the stimulation of naturally occurring 460Id-specific T_s cells can be caused by 460Id-bearing receptors of B cells and/or by small amounts of 460Id-bearing molecules (Bona and Paul, 1979b).

Dohi and Nisonoff (1973) findings favor this explanation with regard to the stimulation of Id-specific T cells.

The target of inhibitory activity of Id-specific T cells seems to be B cells rather than T_h cells. Indeed, Owen *et al.* (1978) have shown that

IdX Ars-specific T_s cells from suppressed A/J mice immunized with KLH-Ars were as effective in adoptive transfer experiments in recipients immunized with KLH-Ars, Edestin-Ars, and HGG-Ars. Interestingly, Id-specific T_s cells which have been very active in the primary response exhibited a weak suppressor activity in the secondary response (Owen and Nisonoff, 1978).

In summary, these data indicated that anti-Id antibodies can generate T_s cells which exert their effects on Id^+ components of antibody response. These findings also indicated that the suppression mediated by T_s cells is idiotype-restricted.

VII. Unresponsiveness of T Cells Induced by Anti-Id Antibodies

Because Id determinants are expressed on the receptor of T and B lymphocytes, the anti-Id antibodies can profoundly alter the function of both lymphocyte subpopulations.

Anti-Id antibodies can suppress the synthesis of Id^+-bearing antibodies either by direct suppression of the precursor or antibody-forming cells or by generation of T_s cells. Similarly, the anti-Id antibodies can suppress the cell-mediated immune responses by T cells.

Thus, the studies of Binz and Wigzell documented the concept that the anti-Id immunity state specific for Id determinants of alloantigen-binding receptor of T cells leads to the unresponsiveness of T cells with respect to their ability to proliferate in MLC, to kill the allogenic target cells, or to mediate GVH or allograft rejection reactions.

The anti-Id immunity was obtained by immunization of mice with syngeneic blast T cells purified from MLC cultures. The anti-Id antibodies obtained after such immunization exhibited the same specificity as anti-Id antibodies obtained by the immunization with alloantibodies.

For example, the mice of A strain have been immunized with A anti-B blast T cells. The anti-Id antibodies produced by A strain subsequent to immunization with A anti-B T blasts were similar to the anti-Id antibodies produced following immunization with A anti-B alloantibodies.

Andersson *et al.* (1977) have shown that the MLC and cytotoxic reactivity of T cells originating from mice with anti-Id immunity was strongly inhibited compared to the control T lymphocytes. Similar results were obtained in rats and guinea pigs, indicating that the unresponsiveness of T cells of animals with anti-Id immunity is a general phenomenon.

Aguet *et al.* (1978) have shown that GVH reactions could be inhibited in the mice and rats with anti-Id immunity specific for Id determinants of the receptor of T cells for alloantigens. In these experiments a direct relationship was observed between the concentration of anti-Id antibodies and the resistance to GVH reaction.

Stuart *et al.* (1976) have studied the survival of kidney allograft in the rats with anti-Id immunity. In this experimental protocol the anti-Id antibodies have been obtained in Lewis rats injected with Lewis anti-BN alloantiserum.

The survivial of LBN F_1 allograft was considerably prolonged, and the GVH reaction upon injection of LBN F_1 cells was prevented. The resistance to allograft and GVH reactions was paralleled with a decrease of MLC and cytotoxic reactivity of T cells in the recipient rats.

Binz and Wigzell (1978) have studied the mechanisms of unresponsiveness of T cells in the hosts with anti-Id immunity. They found that the animals with anti-Id immunity have autoanti-Id killer cells which probably eliminate the effector T cells of various cell-mediated immune responses. In their system C57BL/6 mice have been immunized with C57BL/6 anti-CBA T blasts. The lymphocytes from these mice did not proliferate in the presence of CBA-stimulating cells and did not exhibit a cytotoxic activity.

Interestingly, the T cells from these mice were cytotoxic against the syngeneic C57BL/6 anti-CBA T blasts which have been used as immunogens to induce the anti-Id immunity. The specificity of these cytotoxic T cells was proved by their inability to kill C57BL/6 anti-DBA/2 or CBA anti-C57BL/6 T blasts.

The conclusion of these experiments was that the hosts with anti-Id immunity developed autoanti-Id killer cells which eliminated the effector cells bearing Id determinants and thus led to the unresponsiveness of T cells to alloantigens. This unresponsiveness state can be transferred in mildly irradiated mice by Lyt $1^-2^+3^+$ cells and in a lesser degree with Lyt $1^+2^-3^-$ cells.

The results of these observations indicated that the unresponsiveness of T cells in the host with anti-Id immunity represent an active phenomenon which is related to the occurrence of autoanti-Id killer cells responsible of the suppression of various effector T cell subsets.

6

Immune Network: Regulation of Lymphocyte Functions by Anti-idiotype Antibodies

The production of antibody molecules is a complex phenomenon which is genetically programmed and restricted, and which is under the control of various feedback positive or negative mechanisms mediated by cells or by antibody.

The clonal theory (Burnet, 1959) provided a satisfactory explanation of the specificity of the immune response, but this theory considered that the immune apparatus is constituted by independent clones which interact only with foreign antigens. The receptor of lymphocytes recognizes mainly nonself components of the antigenic dictionary, since the clones reactive to self antigens are deleted during ontogeny. However, the clonal theory does not encompass recent observations such as self-recognition within the immune system and the interaction between T and B clones which cooperate in a particular immune response, since the same set of V region genes encode the specificity of their receptor for antigen and the genetic restriction of the collaboration between T, B, and accessory cells. The self recognition process operates at both T cell and antibody level.

The T cell should interact with antigens as well as with self structures encoded by MHC to provide efficient help during a humoral or cell-mediated immune response. Antibody molecules interact with antigens but also with anti antibodies specific for isotypic, allotypic, and idiotypic determinants of Ig molecule.

If there are very few isotypic and allotypic determinants on an Ig molecule of one individual and the animals are highly tolerant to them, the number of Id determinants that an animal is able to produce is very high (Kunkel, 1970). In addition, Id determinants are immunogenic and can elicit both the production of anti-Id autoantibodies and the occurrence of the idiotype specific helper, suppressor, or effector (i.e., killer) T cells.

Therefore, another aspect of the regulation of the immune response which was not encompassed by clonal theory was the regulation of clonal expression by anti-Id antibodies or idiotype-specific T cells. The hypothesis of Jerne (1974, 1976) which considered the immune system as a web of V domains suggested the possibility of a self-regulatory mechanism of the immune system through idiotype–anti-idiotype interactions.

I. Network Concept

The network theory emerged from several important data which have been accumulated during the last 10 years. The most important finding is the dual character of antibody molecule which is able to combine specifically with antigens but is antigenic itself by virtue of the immunogenicity of its antigenic determinants. The idiotypic determinants of the antibody molecules can elicit an anti-Id autoantibody response during a normal immune response elicited by conventional immunization with a particular antigen. Furthermore, naturally occurring idiotype-specific suppressor T cells which regulate the Id^+ component of an antibody response were also observed. These findings have shown that the repertoire of V domains is constituted by the repertoire of combining sites and the repertoire of idiotypes. Both repertoires are reflected in the receptors of T and B cells. The receptor specific for antigens of T cells shares Id determinants with antibodies specific for the same antigen, whereas the receptor specific for idiotype shares Id determinants of anti-Id antibodies.

The new theoretical approaches to explain the appearance of antibody diversity based on the molecular studies indicated that the repertoire of V region structural genes is large enough to cover the antigenic dictionary provided by nonself and self (including the idiotypes) antigens.

Discovery that the same set of V region genes encoded the specificity of the receptor for antigens of both T and B cells was another important finding which supported the network theory. This indicated that the T and B cell clones can be susceptible to the same immunoregulatory signals represented by anti-Id antibodies. Indeed, numerous findings demonstrated that anti-Id antibodies can regulate the function of T and B lymphocytes. These data also indicated very clearly that after antigenic stimulation the T and B cells do not develop as autonomous, independent clones but that their functions can be modulated by a second degree of interaction of antibody molecules, i.e., between idiotypes and anti-idiotypes.

Idiotype–anti-idiotype interactions provide positive and/or negative immunoregulatory signals and can satisfy the basic regulation requirement of the immune response.

According to network theory the antibody (Ab_1)-bearing Id_1 determinants is able to elicity the synthesis of an anti-Id antibody (Ab_2). This later suppresses the production of Ab_1, but by virtue of its new set of Id determinants (Id_2) can induce the synthesis of Ab_3 and "buffer" other sets of anti-idiotypic antibodies, etc. The basic pattern of network is essentially suppression, since only it can guarantee the maintainence of a steady state, an equilibrium between various components of the network. For a long time it was considered that Id determinants are strictly associated with combining site of antibody molecules; increasing evidence clearly showed that at least two distinct categories of Id determinants can exist. One category is associated with the combining site and another with the framework segments of V region.

Lindemann (1979) makes a distinction between the anti-Id antibodies which interact with combining site of antibody molecules and block the binding of antigen. These antibodies called homobodies represent the internal image of antigens, the positive topochemical copies of the antigen. However, in a network system both Id determinants associated with combining site and with the framework segments can elicit the production of the anti-Id antibodies. These two categories of Id determinants of anti-Id antibodies could in turn elicit the synthesis of other two sets of anti-Id antibodies. It, therefore, appears that network systems can generate a large diversity of anti-Id antibodies in which two parallel sets of molecules specific for the combining site or framework associated Id determinants can coexist (Fig. 6.1).

It might be postulated that the coexistence of these two sets of

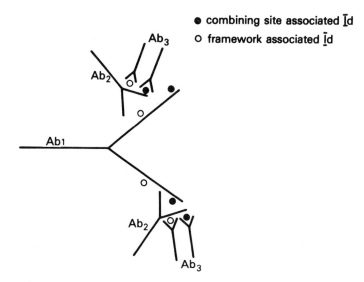

● combining site associated Ĭd
○ framework associated Ĭd

Fig. 6.1. Two sets of anti-idiotypic antibodies which could occur.

populations of anti-Id antibodies lead more easily to the suppression of the antibody (i.e., Ab_1) which triggered the network system. It also clearly appears that each antigen and its corresponding antibody has their particular network system in which the dominance of one or the other set of anti-Id antibodies as well as the number of idiotype–anti-Id reactions could be very different for various antigens. The antigenic challenge is supposed to upset idiotype equilibrium and the subsequent production of antibodies to breakdown the steady state. The increased concentration of antibodies (Ab_1) can stimulate the production of Ab_2, Ab_3, etc. However, in each successive step of idiotype–anti-Id reactions, a degree of damping can occur and for all but for most exhuberant antibody responses the first regulatory reaction between Ab_1 and Ab_2 is probably sufficient. Additional regulatory steps could provide a fine control and, in some circumstances, enhance the immune response or even to activate the silent repertoire.

The results of the interaction between idiotype and anti-idiotype "can be either a depressing or an enhancing effect of lymphocytes displaying these V domains" (Jerne, 1976). The ensuing years have seen various experimental results which confirmed this major prediction of network theory.

Up to now, several mathematical models have been proposed to describe the kinetics of the immune response in a network regulatory system. The aim of these models was to study the kinetics of idiotype–anti-idiotype reactions which explain the transition from a virgin state to a different configuration responsible for the immune state.

Three categories of mathematical models were constructed.

1. Open model of network based on linear nonreciprocal interaction which leads to an expanding configuration (Richter, 1975) (Fig 6.2).

2. Circular or closed model of network based on interaction between small intracyclic cycles (Hiernaux, 1977) (Fig 6.3).

3. Network system based on T–B cell dichotomy of immune apparatus (Hoffmann, 1975) as well as on enhancing or suppressing effects of anti-Id antibodies (Hiernaux and Bona, 1981; Bona et al., 1981).

The mathematical data as well as their experimental correlates were reviewed recently elsewhere (Hiernaux and Bona, 1981; Bona et al., 1981). Mathematical modeling might be useful in understanding the global picture of the immune network in terms of its structure and its regulation.

II. Demonstration of Formal Network

The network theory is based on the assumption that Id determinants are highly immunogenic and that they can elicit an antibody response among the individuals of a species which did not see or have already seen the Id determinants of an antibody molecule. Thus, Ab_1 bearing Id_1 should trigger a chain of complementary anti-Id antibody responses, e.g., Ab_2 bearing Id_2, Ab_3 bearing Id_3, etc., in the same individual.

The possibility of inducing a series of complementary anti-Id responses was demonstrated in the rabbit, which is an outbred species, and in a syngeneic system in BALB/c mice. The results obtained in these experiments suggested that the chain of anti-Id antibody responses can be induced in an experimental system.

In the rabbit Urbain et al. (1977) were able to obtain a series of these complementary anti-Id antibodies (i.e., Ab_2, Ab_3, and Ab_4).

The first rabbit was immunized with Micrococcus lysodeikticus

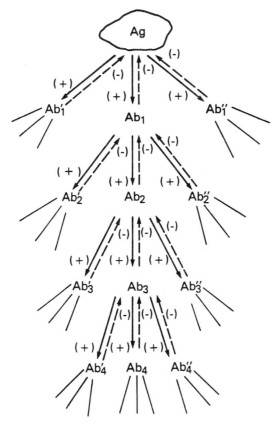

Fig. 6.2. Open idiotypic network. The antigen stimulates the proliferation of various Ab_1, which in turn induce the production of different Ab_2, etc. In such a network, the number of clones involved in the regulation of an immune response grows very rapidly. The arrows correspond to stimulatory processes, and the dashed arrows to suppressive processes.

polysaccharide (CHO), and the anti-CHO antibodies from this rabbit were used in a second unrelated rabbit in order to prepare anti-Id antibodies (i.e., Ab_2). The Ab_2 produced by second rabbit was used as immunogen to prepare anti-(anti-Id) antibodies, i.e., Ab_3, in other unrelated rabbits. Finally, Wikler *et al.* (1979) used Ab_3 to prepare in a fourth unrelated rabbit Ab_4. Cazenave (1977) obtained in unrelated rabbits Ab_2 and Ab_3 in a system in which the Ab_1 was an anti-bovine RNase antibody.

The series of anti-Id antibodies obtained in these experiments

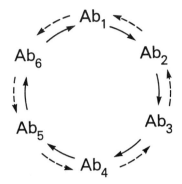

Fig. 6.3. Even cycle of interacting lymphocytes and antibodies of species Ab_1, Ab_2, etc.

seems to be true anti-Id antibodies, since they have been prepared in allotype matched rabbits. In Urbain's experiment a, b, e, c, and d series identical allotype rabbits were used. However, since no information has been provided with regard to the Ig class of Ab_1, Ab_2, and Ab_3 used as immunogens the anti-allotypic contaminants against x and y allotypic determinants of V_H region and of n, f, and g allotypic determinants of $C\mu$ and $C\alpha$ regions, respectively, cannot be completely excluded. In Cazenave's experiment the rabbits used to prepare Ab_1, Ab_2, and Ab_3 have been matched only for a and b series [i.e. they were a ($1^-2^-3^+$) b ($4^+5^-6^-9^-$) phenotype].

Therefore, the immunochemical analysis of the Ab_3 obtained in response to immunization with homologous anti-Id antibodies should take in consideration the exhaustive allotype matching which was carried out in the experiments in which an outbred species is used. However, similar results were obtained in a syngeneic animal system. We used as Ab_1 the DNP-binding MOPC460 myeloma protein of BALB/c origin. Anti-460Id antibodies were prepared in BALB/c mice, and after chromatography affinity purification they were used to prepare in another group of BALB/c mice anti-(anti-Id) antibodies. We have shown that these anti-(anti-460Id) antibodies agglutinated only SRBC coated with anti-460Id antibodies but not with other Ig classes bearing *a* allotype (Bona *et al.*, 1979c). Therefore, it appeared clearly that even in a syngeneic system we can induce a complementary series of anti-Id antibodies.

What is the significance of these results for the existence of a network? The major objection of these experiments is that the series of complementary anti-Id antibodies has been obtained in different individuals of an outbred species or in different groups of syngeneic mice.

Although these results represent a clear, formal demonstration of the network, we do not know the extent of anti-Id antibody responses which can take place *in vivo* in one individual after antigenic stimulation.

However, the immunochemical analysis of Ab_1–Ab_4 suggests that these complementary anti-Id antibody responses could represent a mimicry of the functional network. Urbain *et al.* (1977) and later Wikler *et al.* (1979) have shown that Ab_3 shares Id determinants with anti-CHO antibodies (i.e., Ab_1) and that Ab_4 shares Id determinants with Ab_2.

We have obtained similar results in A48Id system by analyzing the immunochemical properties of four members of a syngeneic network pathway [i.e., A48 (Ab_1), anti-A48Id. (Ab_2), anti-(anti-A48Id) (Ab_3), and anti-[anti-(anti-A48Id)] (Ab_4) antibodies. Our study showed that Ab_1 and Ab_3 share cross-idiotype despite the fact that Ab_3 fails to bind the antigen. The Ab_2 and Ab_4 bind to Ab_1 but the affinity of Ab_4 to Ab_1 is about 300 times lower than that of Ab_2 to Ab_1 (Bona *et al.,* 1981).

The idiotypic similarity between Ab_1 and Ab_3 and, on the other hand, between Ab_2 and Ab_4 suggests strongly a circular network based on interaction between small intercyclic cycles.

The results of mimicry of a functional network in different individuals in syngeneic or outbred animals, have the "potency" to answer the question on which extent the anti-Id antibodies represent the internal image of antigens and the degeneracy of this image during the complementary anti-Id antibody responses. Unfortunately, since only few systems have been investigated the answer is not very clear.

It appears that in three different systems the anti-(anti-Id) antibodies, i.e., Ab_3 do not recognize the antigen which elicited the production of Ab_1. Thus, Urbain *et al.* (1977) have found that Ab_3 does not recognize CHO antigen. Cazenave (1977) showed that Ab_3 does not interact with RNase, and we have found that adsorbtion of anti-(anti-460Id) antibodies on TNP-coupled to Sepharose 4B did not alter the titer of Ab_3. By contrast Wikler *et al.* (1979) observed a striking similarity between Ab_2 and Ab_4 since both sets of anti-Id antibodies recognize Ab_1.

We have found that in some circumstances Ab_3 can recognize the antigen. Roland prepared a series of anti-Id antibodies starting with rabbit b6-bearing Ig as antigen. Anti-b6 allotype antibodies represented in this system Ab_1, anti-(anti-allotype b6 antibodies) the Ab_2 and anti-anti-(anti-allotype b6 antibodies) the Ab_3.

From the radioimmunoassay (RIA) and immunochemical data it was not clear if the Ab_3 interacted with b6 bearing Ig or the rabbit immunized with Ab_2 (i.e. anti-anti-allotype) antibodies elicited the production of Ab_3 which in turn activates the clones able to make anti-allotype antibodies as we have demonstrated that is the case in 460Id system (Bona *et al.*, 1979c).

In this system anti-(anti-460Id) antibodies enhanced 460-Id$^+$ anti-TNP response. Since the RIA assay is too sensitive to discriminate between high amounts of Ab_3 and minute amounts of the putative Ab_1, we decided to test the ability of Ab_3 to induce a blast response. It is known that in rabbit the anti-allotype antibodies which interact with allotype bearing receptors of lymphocytes induce their proliferation and stimulate [^{3}H] thymidine incorporation (Sell and Gell, 1965).

We took advantage of this technique in which the blast response cannot be induced by small amounts of anti-allotypic antibodies. In our experiments a significant increase of [^{3}H]thymidine incorporation was obtained with 50 or 100 μg of Ig fraction of anti-allotype antibodies. Lymphocytes from heterozygous b4/b6 rabbits were incubated with (a) anti-b4 or anti-b6 anti-allotype antibodies (Ab_1), (b) anti-(anti-b6 allotype) antibodies, i.e., Ab_2, and (c) anti-anti-(anti-b6 allotype) antibodies, i.e., Ab_3. Anti-b6 Ab_1 and and Ab_3 antibodies stimulated the incorporation of [^{3}H]thymidine, whereas Ab_2 did not. It should be mentioned that at equal amounts of Ab_1 and Ab_3 the level of incorporated [^{3}H]thymidine was similar.

Therefore, we can conclude from these results (Table 6.1) that Ab_3 and Ab_1 interacted with b6 bearing Ig receptor and caused the blast response. However, we cannot exclude formally that Ab_3 is contaminated with "super" anti-allotype antibody molecules with an extraordinary and unusual affinity and blastogenic ability (Bona *et al.*, 1981).

These findings taken together indicate that we do not have a clear answer to the one important prediction of network theory, namely, if anti-Id antibodies represent the internal image of antigen or not.

However, the idiotypic similarity between Ab_1 and Ab_3 and between Ab_2 and Ab_4 suggests that the diversity of the repertoire does not increase at each step of the complementary anti-Id antibody response. For these reasons we suggested that in each successive step of idiotype–anti-idiotype regulation very substantial degrees of "damping" occur and that for all but most exuberant antibody responses the

TABLE 6.1

[³H]Thymidine Incorporation of Rabbit b4/b6 Lymphocytes Induced by Ammonium Sulfate Fraction of Various Anti-allotype and Anti-idiotype Antisera[a]

b4/b6 rabbit lymphocytes incubated with	cpm ± SD	Stimulation index
—	168 ± 17	—
NWSM, 50 μg/ml	1322 ± 302	7.9
Anti-b4 allotype antibodies[b]		
50 μg/ml	1187 ± 171	7.1
100 μg/ml	1677 ± 191	10.0
Anti-b6 allotype antibodies[c]		
50 μg/ml	928 ± 105	5.5
100 μg/ml	725 ± 168	4.3
Anti-Id specific for anti-b6 allotype antibodies (AB2)[c]		
50 μg/ml	256 ± 86	1.5
100 μg/ml	432 ± 57	2.6
Anti (anti-Id) antibodies (AB3)[c]		
50 μg/ml	848 ± 65	5.0
100 μg/ml	787 ± 55	4.7
Anti-alkaline phosphatase antibodies[c]		
50 μg/ml	141 ± 17	<1
100 μg/ml	132 ± 26	<1

[a] Peripheral blood lymphocytes (2×10^5) were incubated without serum for 48 hours. From Bona *et al.*, 1979c.

[b] Antiserum raised in b5/b6 rabbits.

[c] Antiserum raised in b4/b4 rabbits.

first level of regulatory interaction is probably sufficient. Additional regulatory steps as the occurrence of Ab_3, Ab_4, etc., could provide a fine control of the antibody responses (Bona *et al.*, 1979c).

III. From Formal Network to Functional Network

Numerous experimental findings suggested that the conception of formal network leads to a functional network theory of the regulation of the immune response. The existence of a functional network is supported by two lines of evidence: (1) existence of anti-Id autoantibodies and (2) the ability of anti-Id antibodies to mimic the antigen.

Anti-idiotypic autoantibodies have been observed after intentional immunization as well as spontaneously during the immune responses elicited by conventional antigens. Rodkey (1974) immunized outbred rabbits with p-aminophenyl N-trimethylammonium chloride (TMA)-KLH conjugate and collected sera for 180 days. The anti-TMA antibodies purified by affinity chromatography were injected then into the same rabbit that synthesized antibodies.

These rabbits made an anti-Id autoantibody. The reaction between the anti-Id autoantibody and anti-TMA antibodies was inhibitable with hapten. This experiment clearly demonstrated that one individual is able to synthesize antibodies specific for its own V region and represented the first finding indicating the existence of a network. This idea has been strengthened by experiments which showed the occurrence of anti-Id antibodies during a normal immune response induced by conventional antigens. The results of these experiments will be presented in the next section.

In Chapters 4 and 5 we have described various experimental systems in which it appears that anti-Id antibodies can mimic the function of antigens. In summary, these findings showed that anti-Id antibodies can prime the B cells and induce their maturation in antibody secreting cells (Trenkner and Riblet, 1975; Eichmann and Rajewsky 1975; Bona, 1979a). With regard to the T cells, it was also shown that anti-Id antibodies can stimulate the proliferation of T cells reactive to alloantigen in the absence of antigens (Binz *et al.*, 1979c), can prime the helper T cells (Eichmann and Rajewsky, 1975; Cosenza *et al.*, 1977), and can generate suppressor T cells (Eichmann, 1974; Nisonoff *et al.*, 1977). These observations taken collectively support ideas of a network regulatory mechanism of humoral and cell mediated immune responses.

Various observations and experimental findings indicate that two general types of functional networks exist: suppressive and enhancing networks (Bona, 1979b). These two types of network regulatory mechanisms fit to Jerne's prediction, which considered that anti-Id antibodies could lead either to the suppression or enhancement of the function of lymphocytes.

IV. Suppressive Types of Networks

Hart *et al.* (1972) have shown that the parenteral administration of heterologous anti-Id antibodies leads to the idiotype suppression in adult animals. Intentionally induced idiotype suppression was then obtained in various experimental systems. Later, several investigators observed the presence of anti-Id autoantibodies during a normal immune response induced by a conventional immunization. These observations are highly relevant for a functional network since they demonstrated the autoimmunogenic capacity of Id determinants of antibody molecules as well as their regulatory function. Anti-Id autoantibodies have been detected in the serum by hemagglutination (HA) or RIA assays and at cellular level by PFC or antigen binding cell assays. Anti-Id autoantibodies have been observed in various species.

A. Humoral Anti-Id Autoantibodies

Circulating anti-Id autoantibodies detected by HA or RIA have been observed in various antigenic systems and mammalian species.

1. Phosphocholine (PC)

Kluskens and Kohler (1974) studied the kinetics of the anti-PC-PFC response in BALB/c mice repeatedly immunized with *Pneumococcus* R36A vaccine. In this study, a decrease of anti-PC-PFC response was observed after several immunizations. It seems that this decrease was related to the occurrence of anti-T15Id antibodies. Indeed, it was shown that the sera from BALB/c mice immunized four to five times with *Pneumococcus* R36A vaccine contained hemagglutinins for T15 coated SRBC. Such anti Id autoantibodies were not found in the preimmune sera indicating that T15 anti-PC antibodies produced during the PC response caused their synthesis.

2. Dinitrophenyl-Trinitrophenyl (DNP-TNP)

MOPC 315 and MOPC460 myeloma proteins bind TNP and DNP. The Id determinants of these myeloma proteins are expressed on the anti-TNP and anti-DNP antibodies produced by BALB/c mice in response to immunization with T-independent or T-dependent TNP conjugates (Granato *et al.*, 1974; Bona and Paul, 1979a; Zeldis *et al.*, 1979; Le Guern *et al.*, 1979; Cazenave *et al.*, 1980).

Sirisinha and Eisen (1971) have shown that BALB/c mice immunized with these myeloma proteins develop an anti-315Id or -460Id antibody response which was considered (Eisen *et al.*, 1975) as an autoanti-Id response since both myeloma proteins are of BALB/c origin.

Granato *et al.* (1974) have also observed that BALB/c mice immunized with MOPC315 showed high titers of anti-315Id antibodies. When these mice have been immunized with DNP-KLH, the anti-DNP antibody response was significantly depressed as compared to the normal BALB/c mice. In addition, 315Id bearing anti-TNP antibodies were not detected in the mice preimmunized with MOPC315. Normal BALB/c mice made 315-Id$^+$ anti-DNP antibodies following immunization with DNP-KLH. Similarly, we observed that BALB/c mice immunized with TNP-BL or TNP-NWSM develop a vigorous anti-TNP-PFC response. About 30% of the anti-TNP PFC expressed 460Id. BALB/c immunized with MOPC460 develop anti-460Id antibodies and anti-460Id PFC (Table 6.2). When the mice immunized with MOPC460 have been then immunized with TNP-NWSM, no 460Id anti-TNP secreting PFC were observed. Thus the presence of circulating anti-460Id antibodies and anti-460Id PFC seems to be responsible for the failure of these mice to develop 460Id anti-TNP-PFC response.

3. *Micrococcus lysodeikticus* Polysaccharide (PS)

Brown *et al.* (1979) have studied in the rabbits the kinetics of anti-PS response as well as the clonotype pattern during a 31-month period in which the rabbits were immunized three times with *Micrococcus lysodeikticus* polysaccharide. After the first immunization only a strong anti-PS response was observed. After the second immunization the simultaneous presence of anti-PS and anti-Id antibodies was observed. After the third immunization the anti-Id antibodies were not detected.

These isoelectric focusing analyses of clonotype patterns provided interesting data. Thus some clonotypes observed after first immunization were absent or were reduced in quantity after the second immunization when anti-Id autoantibodies had occurred. During the period of the anti-Id antibody synthesis new clonotypes were also detected.

Finally, after the third immunization, which was devoid of detectable anti-Id autoantibodies, the clonotypes observed after first immunization and those which emerged after the second immunization were observed together. This elegant observation clearly shows that some Id bearing anti-PS antibodies elicited the synthesis of anti-Id antibodies. These anti-Id antibodies had a double regulatory effect:

TABLE 6.2

Anti-idiotypic Antibody Response to MOPC460 by BALB/c Mice

Hemagglutinin response (n = 12)		PFC response (n = 5)			Specificity of anti-460 Id PFC		
			PFC/10^7 spleen cells				Direct anti-MOPC460 PFC/10^7 spleen cells
SRBC coated with	HA titer (ln)	SRBC coated with	Direct	Indirect	Inhibitor	Amount (µg)	
MOPC460	5.83 ± 0.68	MOPC460	61.3 ± 15.5	15.8 ± 3.6	None	—	147 ± 9
MOPC167	0	U-61	3.3 ± 3.3	6.0 ± 2.8	MOPC460	1	89 ± 7
						10	30 ± 3
						100	15 ± 4
					U61	1	148 ± 13
						10	141 ± 11
						100	81 ± 13

they exerted a reversible inhibitory effect on some clones and favored the expression of silent clones.

4. Anti-alloantigen Response

McKearn *et al.* (1974) have prepared in F_1 rats (Lewis × Brown Norway) an anti-Id antibody directed against Lewis anti-BN alloimmune serum. These anti-Id antisera recognize Lewis anti-BN antibodies from several individuals indicating that it interacted with an IdX expressed on these anti-alloantigen sera. Surprisingly, the authors did not find IdX bearing anti-alloantigen antibodies in Lewis rats immunized six times with BN cells. However, they have found that the sera of these hyperimmunized rats contain anti-Id autoantibodies. The rats having anti-Id autoantibodies lacked IdX bearing anti-BN antigen antibodies.

5. Anti-allotype Response

Recently we have reported that anti-allotype antibodies specific for *b* allelic form of IgG_{2a} produced in various strains of mice expressed an IdX. The expression of this IdX is independent of various genetic markers such as H-2, Igh-C (Bona *et al.*, 1980b). We have studied the ability of maternally allotype suppressed (IgG_{2a}^b) F_1 hybrids to make anti-allotype antibodies. In these experiments the allotype suppression was obtained in F_1 hybrids prepared by mating of BALB/c female mice immunized with CBPC101 myeloma protein (IgG_{2a}^b) with C.B20 male mice. At 3 months, 22 out of 24 F_1 hybrids failed to express the paternal allotype (IgG_{2a}^b of C.B20 male mice) and did not have detectable hemagglutinins against CBPC101 from the mother. The mice immunized with CBPC101 myeloma protein made a low but significant titer of anti-allotype antibodies. Surprisingly, these anti-allotype antibodies lacked IdX (Table 6.3).

In RIA we observed that the sera of these mice used as inhibitors caused actually a stronger binding of labeled anti-allotype antibodies to microplates coated with anti-IdX antibodies. Therefore, we have tested in direct assay the ability of the sera of suppressed mice to bind labeled anti-allotype antibody. We have found that the sera from a majority of mice bound the labeled anti-IgG_{2a}^b allotype antibodies (Table 6.4). These results strongly suggested that the inability of these mice to develop an IdX^+ anti-allotype response was related to the spontaneous occurrence of anti-IdX antibodies (Bona, 1980b). These

TABLE 6.3

Absence of IdX on Anti-(IgG$_{2a}^{b}$) Allotype Antibodies Produced by Maternally Allotype-Suppressed (BALB/c × C.B210)F$_1$ Mice Immunized with CBPC101 Myeloma Protein[a]

F$_1$ No.	HA titer (ln)			HI titer (ln)	
	CBPC101	C57BL/6 Ig	UPC10	BAB14 anti-Id	CXB1 anti-Id
1	0	0	0	0	0
2	5	5	0	0	0
3	5	5	0	0	0
4	5	5	0	0	0
5	2	2	0	0	0
7	5	5	0	0	0
8	3	3	0	0	0
9	3	4	0	0	0
10	6	6	0	0	0
11	4	4	0	0	0
12	6	5	0	0	0
13	4	4	0	0	0
15	4	5	0	0	0
16	5	5	0	0	0
17	4	5	0	0	0
18	2	1	0	0	0
19	5	4	0	0	0
20	5	0	0	0	0
21	5	4	0	0	0
22	3	5	0	0	0
23	4	5	0	0	0
24	1	1	0	0	0

[a] From Bona, 1980b.

anti-Id autoantibodies suppressed the IdX$^+$ component of the anti-allotype antibodies.

B. Serum Inhibitory Factors Behaving as Anti-Id Antibodies

In several antigenic systems, it was observed that the sera from immune animals contain inhibitory factors of antibody secreting or binding cells which have been considered to be anti-Id antibodies. In general these experiments did not provide immunochemical informa-

TABLE 6.4

Binding of ^{3}H-Labeled BALB/c Anti-CBPC101 Antibodies to BAB.14 Anti-Idiotypic Serum and to Spontaneous Anti-idiotypic Autoantibodies Produced by Maternally Allotype-Suppressed (BALB/c × C.B20)F$_1$ Hybrids Immunized with CBPC101 Myeloma Protein[a]

Origin of serum	No. of mice	Binding of ^{3}H-labeled BALB/c anti-CBPC101[b] antibody to microplates coated with various sera
BAB 14 anti-Id serum (diluted 5 × 10^{-4})	Pool	2560[c]
BAB 14 normal serum (diluted 5 × 10^{-4})	Pool	103
BALB/c normal serum (diluted 1:10)	Pool	87
Serum from nonimmunized maternally suppressed F$_1$ hybrids (diluted 1:2)	10	350[d], 283, 275, 252, 258, 211, 183, 122, 118, 98
Serum from maternally suppressed F$_1$ hybrids immunized with myeloma proteins	19	2510[c], 2150, 1835, 1132[f], 1637, 935, 1675, 1501, 1487, 756, 736, 831, 830, 1408, 1395, 1291, 812, 805, 799, 795, 1187, 1185, 1184, 786, 603, 601, 592, 1073, 1052, 856, 556, 570, 534, 490 833, 720, 710, 650

[a] From Bona, 1980b.
[b] 15,000 cpm of ^{3}H-labeled BALB/c anti-CBPC101 was added for each well.
[c] Counts per minute.
[d] Each represents an individual mouse tested.
[e] These values are for sera diluted 1:2.
[f] These values are for sera diluted 1:8.

tion about the Id determinants of antibodies with which these putative anti-Id antibodies interact.

Bankert and Pressman (1976) studied the ability of sera from rabbits immunized with SRBC or NIP conjugate to inhibit the antigen binding capacity of lymph node lymphocytes. The rationale behind these experiments followed other data which showed that anti-receptor antibodies which can occur spontaneously during the immune response can block the antigen binding cells. Indeed, 7-day serum harvested from rabbits immunized with SRBC or NIP inhibited the antigen-binding capacity of lymphocytes from immune rabbits. This inhibitory factor looked like an anti-Id idiotype since in that it was an IgG, and was specific. The serum from rabbits immunized with SRBC did not inhibit NIP-binding cells. In addition, the serum from rabbit A inhibited 34% of antigen binding cells of rabbit A and only 3% of rabbit B. Inhibitory activity never exceeded 64% indicating that anti-Id autoantibodies have been produced only against the Id determinants expressed on certain clones. These data strongly supported the idea that the serum inhibitory factor was an anti-Id antibody.

A putative anti-Id antibody responsible for the rapid decline of anti-TNP-PFC response in AKR mice following immunization with TNP-Ficoll was reported by Schrater et al. (1979a). Their data are in agreement with that previously reported which showed that anti-315- and 460Id antibodies produced in BALB/c mice subsequent to active immunization ablated the 315Id and 460Id positive component of the anti-TNP antibody response. Schrater et al. (1979b) have shown that the anti-TNP-PFC response declines between days 4 and 7 after immunization with TNP-Ficoll. In these experiments it was shown that the decline of the anti-TNP-PFC response between days 4 and 7 was only apparent since the number of these plaques can be increased by the addition into agarose of the free hapten (TNP-EACA). It was suggested that the hapten caused the displacement of the putative anti-Id antibody from the surface of cells secreting anti-TNP antibodies. These anti-Id antibodies could be found in the sera of BALB/c mice. Indeed these sera injected in normal BALB/c mice accelerated the appearance of hapten augmentable anti-TNP-PFC.

In this study no immunochemical characterization of anti-Id antibody and of Id borne by anti-TNP antibodies was provided as was done in 315Id and 460Id anti-TNP system. However, Goidl et al. (1979) provided some suggestive data indicating that the inhibitor factor responsible of the decline of anti-TNP-PFC response could be an anti-Id antibody.

This inhibitory activity can be removed by an anti-mouse Ig and AKR anti-TNP autoantibody immunoadsorbants. By contrast, this inhibitory activity was not affected by passage over columns coated with rabbit anti-TNP, AKR anti-dansyl antibodies, or TNP-BSA.

The decline of the anti-TNP antibody response was explained therefore by the appearance of cells which secrete anti-Id antibodies which in turn block the secretion process of anti-TNP antibody forming cells.

Two experimental findings favored this explanation.

1. The suppression of the anti-TNP response was transferable by B cells from 7 day immunized BALB/c mice injected into normal mice.

2. The putative anti-Id antibody was eluted with hapten from the surface of 7 day immune spleen cells. However, the experimental verification of this proposed mechanism can be provided by a crucial experiment in which it can be shown that anti-TNP antibodies prepared from 2-day immune serum can induce the synthesis of anti-Id antibodies in normal AKR mice by day 5.

$\alpha(1\rightarrow6)$ Dextran

Fernandez *et al.* (1979) have observed that the sera from CBA or C57BL/6 mice harvested 8–14 days after a primary immunization with dextran B512 [i.e., $\alpha(1\rightarrow6)$] was able to suppress the anti-$\alpha(1\rightarrow6)$dextran PFC response.

This inhibitory activity of the sera was not due either to antigen, since the treatment with dextrinase did not affect the inhibitory capacity, or to anti-dextran antibodies, since the sera were extensively adsorbed on Sephadex beads.

Most probably, the inhibition of anti-$\alpha(1\rightarrow6)$dextran PFC by these sera was due to spontaneously occurring anti-Id autoantibodies; these antibodies can be responsible for the decline of anti-dextran response as well as for the failure of these strains to develop a secondary immune response. Interestingly, the inhibition of anti-$\alpha(1\rightarrow6)$dextran PFC was observed only with serum from allotypically identical mice. Thus, the CBA serum inhibited only the PFC of CBA and C_3HT_1f mice but not of C57BL/6 and CBA/Ig-1^b. By contrast the C57BL/6 serum inhibited the PFC of C57BL/6 and CBA/Ig-1^b mice but does not inhibit the PFC of CBA or C_3HT_1f mice.

These results suggested that these anti-idiotypic autoantibodies recognized Id determinants of anti-$\alpha(1\rightarrow6)$dextran antibodies which are under the control of *Igh-C* genes.

In summary, the data reported above clearly showed that in various antigenic systems and in various animal species the anti-Id autoantibodies can be detected in the sera of immune animals and that these antibodies exert a suppressive type of regulatory effect on Id$^+$ components of a given antibody response.

C. Auto Anti-Id Plaque Forming Cells

Support for the functional network also comes from the demonstration of plaque forming cells specific for T15 and E109 idiotypes which occur spontaneously in BALB/c mice immunized with bacterial levan (BL) or phosphocholine (PC). Cosenza (1976) have studied the kinetics of the anti-PC and anti-T15 PFC responses after the priming of BALB/c mice with R36A vaccine. He scored the number of anti-PC and anti-T15 PFC in the same group of BALB/c mice sacrificed at various intervals after immunization. The number of anti-PC-PFC increased 1 day after immunization, reached the peak by day 4, and started to decline by day 8. The auto anti-T15Id PFC were detected by day 6 and reached the peak by day 8 when the anti-PC-PFC started to decline.

Similarly, we observed that the cyclic pattern of anti-BL and -inulin response corresponded to a decrease of E109 Id positive component of anti-BL and anti-inulin PFC responses. In addition, the decline of IdX components of these responses coincided with the occurrence of direct and indirect anti-E109 PFC (Bona *et al.,* 1978).

These two observations strongly suggest that anti-Id antibodies produced during the normal immune response exert their suppressive effects on Id bearing antibody forming cells. Thus, the cyclic pattern is not related to a simple clearing of Id bearing molecules by anti-idiotypic autoantibodies and is due to a true inhibition of cells which secrete Id bearing antibodies.

D. Idiotype Binding Cells

Another approach to study the occurrence of an anti-Id antibody response was to investigate the appearance of cells which bind Id bearing antibodies. The rationale of this approach was that the synthesis of anti-Id antibodies should be paralleled at the cellular level by the occurrence of cells bearing anti-Id receptor.

Tasiaux *et al.* (1978) studied in rabbits immunized with tabacco mosaic virus (TMV) the presence of cells which bind anti-TMV antibodies. Such cells were detected by incubation of peripheral blood lymphocytes from immune rabbits with fluoresceinated anti-TMV antibodies isolated from the cearly phase of the immune response.

About 1% of lymphocytes bound anti-TMV antibodies after the first injection with TMV. After the second injection the number of cells which bind anti-TMV antibodies has fallen to the background level, and they reached the level of 1% after a few months.

Cells able to bind anti-TMV antibodies were found in both T and B lymphocyte subpopulations. A striking correlation was observed between the appearance of anti-Id lymphocytes and the decrease of the affinity of anti-TMV antibodies.

A similar method was used by Jackson and Mestecky (1979) to study in the rabbits the plasma cells which possess the ability to bind anti-human serum albumin (HSA) antibodies. In this study the lymphocytes from rabbits immunized with HSA have the ability to bind autologous, homologous, and even heterologous anti-HSA antibodies, indicating that the receptor of these cells was specific for an IdX of anti-HSA antibodies. The percentage of cells which bound the anti-HSA antibodies depends on the duration of the immunization. A certain variability of the number of Id binding cells was observed among individuals. This variability can be due to the degree of the receptor of anti-Id cells to interact with the IdX expressed on anti-HSA antibodies.

Kelsoe and Cerny (1979) have used the same method to study the anti-T15 binding cells during the primary response of BALB/c mice immunized with R36A vaccine. They studied in parallel the number of anti-PC-PFC. In this study, it was observed that the anti-PC-PFC response peaked at days 2, 10, and 14, and the number of T15 binding cells at days 4 and 12.

In these three mentioned studies, adequate controls of the Id binding cells have been performed. These cells do not bind antibodies which express an unrelated idiotype. Despite the invaluable information provided by these studies, the method of enumeration of Id binding cells can be the subject of a major objection.

It is possible that the antigen associated firmly with the membrane or internalized into the cells can persist for a long time during the immune response and cannot be easily washed out. If it is so, this cell-associated antigen can bind the fluoresceinated antibodies, and this binding would account for scoring the antigen-binding cells and not the cells with receptors specific for idiotypes. Thus, in Kelsoe *et al.* (1980) experiments T15 binding lymphocytes have been found in nude mice despite the fact that these mice cannot make anti-Id antibodies.

However, the presence of anti-Id autoantibodies in the serum as well as auto anti-Id PFC strongly suggests that the anti-Id autoantibodies occur spontaneously during a conventional immune response. The cyclic pattern of immune responses in which anti-Id autoantibodies have been observed and the inverse fluctuation between the Id component of the antibody response clearly indicates the regu-

latory role of the anti-Id antibodies. In fact, a triple relationship between antigens, antibodies, and anti-Id antibodies appears to exist.
The antigens induced the production of antibodies which express a
particular idiotype. When the idiotype bearing antibodies reach a critical level they induce the synthesis of anti-Id antibodies which in turn
suppress the activity of IdX bearing antibody secreting cells.

The appearance of anti-Id autoantibody response needs T cells.
Janneway (1975) has clearly shown that the mice immunized with
myeloma proteins generated helper T cells which have been specific
for idiotypes.

In our study of the kinetics of anti-inulin and anti-bacterial levan
antibody responses we have found a cyclic pattern in normal BALB/c
mice but not in nude BALB/c mice. Furthermore, we have been unable to detect auto anti-E109Id PFC in the nude mice. These results
which suggested that anti-Id autoantibody response is dependent of T
help were supported by two indeptendent studies.

Schrater *et al.* (1979b) have shown that although the nude mice
develop an excellent anti-TNP response, they do not make anti-Id
antibodies. The failure to make anti-Id antibodies explain the slower
decline of the anti-TNP response in nude mice. Similar results were
obtained in Tx mice irradiated and reconstituted with bone marrow.

Similarly, Kelsoe *et al.* (1980) did not observe the cyclic pattern of
anti-PC-PFC in nude mice nor of T15Id binding lymphocytes. In the
nude mice the number of T15 binding lymphocytes was lower than in
normal mice and did not show variations.

It should be mentioned that in the nude mice the magnitude of
anti-BL, anti-TNP, and anti-PC antibody responses was equal and
even higher than in normal BALB/c mice. Therefore, it would seem
that the failure of nude mice to develop anti-Id autoantibodies is not
related to an insufficient idiotypic stimulus but to the absence of the T
cells. This explanation is supported by Kelsoe *et al.* (1980) which
showed that the cyclic pattern of both anti-PC-PFC response and of
T15Id binding cells was restored after graft of the thymus of nude
mice.

V. Enhancing Type of Network

The basic regulatory pattern of the idiotype–anti-Id reaction is suppression. However, it also was shown that anti-Id antibodies can

mimic antigens and therefore, in some circumstances can stimulate the lymphocytes. Similarly, the anti-(anti-Id) antibodies can enhance the immune response.

Urbain *et al.* (1977) and Cazenave (1977) have shown that anti-(anti-Id) antibodies (i.e., Ab_3) stimulated the expression of some silent clones. In these experiments anti-CHO and anti-RNase antibodies (i.e., Ab_1) were prepared from a single rabbit. These antibodies were used as immunogens to induce production of anti-Id antibodies in a second rabbit. These Ab_2 antibodies were used to produce anti-(anti-Id) antibodies (i.e., Ab_3) in the third group of normal rabbits. Interestingly, when these rabbits were immunized with CHO or RNase, they made Ab_1 which expressed the Id determinants of Ab_1 produced by unrelated rabbits. We concluded from these results that anti-(anti-Id) antibodies activated silent clones of the repertoire of unrelated rabbits. However, the activation of silent clones raised several questions: (1) What is the mechanism which maintains the silent clones suppressed? (2) How are the silent clones activated by anti-(anti-Id) antibodies? (3) What is the relationship between anti-Id or anti-(anti-Id) antibodies and the cells which express idiotypes or are specific for idiotypes.

We have tried to answer these questions by studying the cellular basis of expression of idiotypes in the network system. We have chosen as model the $460Id^+$ component of anti-TNP response since we succeeded in preparing syngeneic anti-(anti-460Id) antibodies. We have found that in BALB/c mice after immunization with TNP-levan (TNP-BL), TNP-dextran (TNP-DX), and TNP-*Nocardia* water-soluble mitogen (TNP-NWSM), 10–25% of anti-TNP-PFC secreted antibodies expressing 460Id.

Molecules bearing 460Id were found only in the sera of immune animals and not in the preimmune sera by RIA using as ligand a labeled monoclonal anti-460Id antibody. A similar percentage of 460Id anti-TNP-PFC was observed after *in vitro* stimulation of BALB/c spleen cells with TNP-NWSM. Interestingly, the proportion of $460Id^+$ anti-TNP-PFC was substantially increased when the T cells have been eliminated subsequent to pretreatment with anti-Thy-1.2 serum + C. Furthermore, the addition of T cells to B cells inhibited the $460Id^+$ component of anti-TNP response. These results indicated that a naturally occurring subset of T cells regulates the expression of $460Id^+$ component of the anti-TNP response.

These T cells were specific for 460Id, since we were able to ablate the suppression activity by incubation in petri dishes coated with

MOPC460 myeloma protein (Bona *et al.*, 1979c). In further experiments we have studied the proportion of 460Id$^+$ components of the anti-TNP antibody response in three groups of BALB/c mice immunized with TNP-BL or TNP-NWSM.

1. In normal mice the 460Id$^+$ component represented a minor fraction of anti-TNP response (10–20%).
2. In BALB/c mice immunized with MOPC460 which showed serum anti-460Id antibodies and anti-460Id PFC, no 460Id$^+$ anti-TNP-PFC have been detected.
3. In BALB/c mice immunized with anti-MOPC460 which made anti-(anti-460Id) antibodies, the 460Id component of the anti-TNP antibodies was substantially increased as assessed by RIA, HI, and PFC assays (Table 6.5). Furthermore, these Ab$_3$ mice lacked 460Id specific suppressor T cells that we have identified both in normal mice and in the mice which made anti-Id antibodies.

Indeed the T cells from Ab$_3$ mice failed to inhibit the 460Id bearing anti-TNP secreting B cells from normal or Ab$_3$ mice: T cells from normal BALB/c inhibited both B cells from normal or Ab$_3$ mice (Ta-

TABLE 6.5

Proportion of Anti-TNP-Antibodies Carrying 460Id in Normal BALB/c and BALB/c Mice Producing Anti-(Anti-460Id) Antibodies (Id-3 Mice)[a]

	TNP-NWSM		TNP-levan	
	Normal	Id-3	Normal	Id-3
Number of mice	5	3	5	4
Anti-TNP PFC/10^6 cells	100 ± 14	84 ± 8	276 ± 15	239 ± 64
Percent 460$^+$	27 ± 12	54 ± 5	12 ± 1	34 ± 5
Anti-levan PFC/10^7 cells	ND[b]	ND	203 ± 130	284 ± 41
Percent E109$^+$	ND	ND	42 ± 5	45 ± 20
Anti-TNP HA titer	6 ± 0.5	8 ± 2	12 ± 0.3	12 ± 0
460-Id HI titer	0.5 ± 0.5	2 ± 1	1 ± 0.5	3.5 ± 0.5
μg 460-Id/ml (RIA)[c]	22 ± 6	57 ± 21	14 ± 6	60 ± 25

[a] Normal BALB/c or Id-3 BALB/c mice were immunized with 30 μg of TNP-NWSM or 50 μg of TNP-levan. These were sacrificed 5 days later and humoral and spleen PFC responses tested. From Bona *et al.*, 1979e.

[b] Not done.

[c] Radioimmunoassay.

TABLE 6.6

Proportion of PFC-Secreting Anti-TNP Antibodies Carrying 460Id in Cultures
of T and B Lymphocytes from Normal and Id-3 BALB/c Mice[a]

Donor of lymphocytes		Anti-TNP-PFC		
B	T	PFC/culture	460-Id[+] PFCE/culture	Percent 460-Id[+] PFC
Normal	—	191 ± 26	73 ± 27	38
Normal	Normal	105 ± 6	12 ± 7	11
Normal	Id-3	134 ± 13	55 ± 13	41
Id-3	—	432 ± 15	224 ± 18	52
Id-3	Normal	440 ± 18	42 ± 26	10
Id-3	Id-3	367 ± 41	206 ± 43	56

[a] B lymphocytes (5×10^5) were cultured alone or with 5×10^5 T lymphocytes in
microtiter wells with 5 μg/ml of TNP-NWSM for 4 days. Anti-TNP PFC in the absence
or presence of BALB/c anti-460 antiserum (1/100 dilution) were measured using
TNP-SRBC. From Bona *et al.*, 1979e.

ble 6.6). Therefore, these results indicated that 460Id specific suppressor T cells were eliminated in Ab₃ BALB/c mice by anti-(anti-Id)
antibodies since they share the Id determinants of anti-460Id antibodies (Bona *et al.*, 1979c).

Several conclusions could be drawn from these studies.

1. A functional network consisting of 460Id bearing B cells and
460Id specific suppressor T cells play an important role in the regulation of anti-TNP response, i.e., of 460Id bearing clones which represent a minor component of the BALB/c anti-TNP repertoire.

2. The anti-(anti-460Id) antibodies enhanced the expression of this
minor clone(s) by eliminating the 460Id specific suppressor T cells.

We have also shown that anti-(anti-Id) antibodies can activate 460Id
clones which are silent in the repertoire of some mice strains
(Cazenave *et al.*, 1980).

The expression of *V* genes which encode 460Id is under the control
of *Igh-C*[a] gene. Therefore, the mice which have other allotypes cannot develop 460Id[+] anti-TNP antibodies. DBA/2 mice which have
Ig-1[c] haplotype cannot make 460Id antibodies after the immunization
with T-dependent or T-independent conjugates. However, DBA/2
mice immunized with monoclonal anti-460Id antibodies made anti-

(anti-460Id) antibodies. When these mice (Ab$_3$) were immunized, the anti-TNP antibodies made by these DBA/2 mice expressed 460Id. From these DBA/2 (Ab$_3$) mice, by cell fusion, we prepared several hybridoma specific for TNP. By radioimmunoassay we were able to show that two of these hybridomas secreted monoclonal anti-TNP antibodies bearing 460Id (Cazenave *et al.* 1980). These results indicated that 460Id bearing clones, which are silent in DBA/2 repertoire, were activated by anti-(anti-460Id) antibodies and that their progeny have been immortalized by cell fusion technique.

Recently we have succeeded in activating in mice another silent clone, namely, A48Id$^+$ antibacterial levan clone through network idiotype manipulations. BALB/c mice, as well as other *Igh-C^a* congenic or recombinant strains of mice, do not express A48Id$^+$ during anti-levan antibody response subsequent to a conventional immunization with soluble bacterial levan or bacterial levan conjugates. However, Hiernaux *et al.* (1981) have found that the pretreatment of 1-day-old BALB/c mice with minute amounts of anti-A48Id antibodies followed by immunization with bacterial levan 1 month later led to a substantial increase of A48Id$^+$ component of anti-levan response. We have also found that adult BALB/c mice which synthesized Ab$_3$ [i.e., anti-(anti-A48Id)] in response to immunization with Ab$_1$ (i.e., A48) or Ab$_2$ (i.e., anti-A48Id) were able to make A48Id antibacterial levan antibodies.

These results indicate that the immune network plays an important role in the regulation of expressed as well as silent clones (Bona, 1981b). In addition, these results suggest that the equilibrium between idiotype and anti-idiotype in nonimmunized animals, as well as during various phases of a conventional immune response is very delicate and can be upset by antigen, idiotype, and anti-idiotype.

However, in our opinion, the network theory as formulated by Jerne and discussed in various mathematical models does not cover new and provoking findings observed during recent years and does not answer some crucial questions.

One of these questions is the maximum extent of an idiotype network in an autologous system. If Ab$_1$, which recognizes the antigen, can initiate an Ab$_2$, Ab$_3$ ... Ab$_n$ chain, it then appears that the immune system is chiefly devoted to the recognition of idiotypes. This can be only true if the idiotypes of Ig molecules represent the topo-chemical copies of epitopes (internal image of the antigen); therefore the antigens are never really completely foreign.

The second finding which cannot be explained by a linear or expanding idiotype–antiidiotype chain, and which appears to be an important feature of the immune network, is the ability of both Ab_2 and Ab_4 to bind to Ab_1. This was clearly demonstrated for two different antigenic systems in rabbits (Wickler *et al.*, 1980) and in mice (Bona *et al.*, 1981). It is possible that among various idiotypes of a particular Ig molecule, which is recognized by a heterologous anti-Id antiserum, only a few idiotypes would function in an autologous system. If so, the idiotype repertoire used as regulatory force within the immune system will be limited to a few idiotypes capable of becoming dominant idiotypes, possibly because it is these determinants that call forth Id-specific T cell regulatory response and anti-Id antibodies.

If in an autologous system only a few idiotypes are immunodominant, this implies that only first step Ab_1–Ab_2 (i.e., idiotype–anti-Id antibody or anti-Id regulatory cells) would be functionally relevant, since Ab_3, Ab_5 ... Ab_{n-1} will be the positive imprints of Ab_1, and Ab_4, Ab_6 ... Ab_n will be the positive imprints of Ab_2.

Studies in progress in various laboratories will certainly provide new data which will contribute to better understanding of the cellular and molecular basis and the genetic control of the idiotype network, as well as to the understanding of the function of the network in autologous systems under various physiological and pathological conditions.

7

Physiological and Pathological Implications of the Immune Network

In an extention of the concept of the regulation of the antibody synthesis and cell-mediated immune responses by the immune network, the regulatory role of antibodies or anti-Id antibodies on the function of nonlymphoid somatic cells became more and more evident.

Several findings suggest that in various neuro- and endocrinopathies the failure of target organs to respond to hormones or transmitters is related to the presence of autoanti-receptor antibodies. The production of the autoantibodies in various autoimmune diseases can be suppressed by anti-Id antibodies. Therefore, there are important therapeutic implications of these findings since several diseases which have been currently treated by injections with hormones or by immunosuppressive agents can be possibly treated by adequate immunological manipulations with anti-Id antibodies.

I. Modulation of Functions of Nonlymphoid Somatic Cells by Antibodies

Mimicry of the functions of hormones or neurotransmitters by antibodies against the receptor of nonlymphoid somatic cells was studied

183

particularly in the case of the receptor for insulin, thyrotropin, and acetylcholine. Antibodies against the receptors which could interfere with hormone activity were also found in other autoimmune diseases, but their role has only recently been documented. Autoantibodies which could block the receptor for hormones can play a role in Addison's disease (i.e., for the receptor for ACTH), pseudohyperparathyroidism (i.e., receptor for parathyroid hormone) and in pernicious anemia (i.e., receptor for gastrin).

A direct interaction between anti-receptor antibody and insulin receptor was demonstrated by immunoprecipitation. Jacobs *et al.* (1978) have prepared a specific antibody in rabbit against the solubilized insulin receptor from rat liver membrane. The antiserum to the receptor mimics the binding of insulin to the receptor. Indeed, it stimulates the conversion of glucose to CO_2 in isolated rat fat cells. Similarly, this antiserum like insulin, inhibited epinephrine-stimulated lipolysis. However, in contrast to insulin, it had little effect on the lipolytic activity. It would be interesting to know whether or not these anti-receptor antibodies can mimic the delayed pharmacological properties of insulin, such as the stimulation of the synthesis of protein and nucleoproteins.

Another example of modulation of function of nonlymphoid somatic cells by anti-receptor antibodies was provided by studies of anti-TSH receptor antibodies. These antibodies were tested with regard to their ability to increase the permeability of thyroid lysosomes and to block the binding of ^{131}I-labeled thyroid-stimulating hormone (TSH) to thyroid membrane.

The increase of the permeability of thyroid lysosomes by TSH accounts for activation of thyroid function subsequent to the binding of TSH to TSH receptor. The increase of this permeability was measured by an increase of the intensity of color of lysosomes after the incubation of thyroid cells with leucyl-β-naphthylamide, which is a chromogenic substrate for a lysosomal enzyme, namely, the leucyl-β-naphthylamidase. The increased uptake of this chromogenic substrate was quantitated by scanning and integrating microfluorometry. IgG anti-TSH antibodies against TSH receptor from three patients with Graves' disease induced a 28.6–38% increase of the uptake of chromogenic substrate by lysosomes of thyroid cells whereas normal IgG induced a 0.4–2.9% increase over the control. The activation of thyroid cell lysosomes by anti-TSH receptor antibodies was paralleled by a blockage of the binding of labeled TSH to thyroid membrane by these antibodies. This blockage was ablated by adsorption of anti-TSH receptor antibodies on thyroid membrane adsorbents (McLachlan *et al.*, 1977). These findings indicate that anti-insulin or TSH receptor antibodies mimic the hormone's activity. By contrast the anti-acetylcholine receptor antibodies accelerate the degradation of the receptor and therefore can alter the function of this neurotransmitter.

Acetylcholine receptor (ACR) is a complex of macromolecules which contain at least two functional constituents: (1) the cation-specific channel and (2) the binding site for acetylcholine. Four glycoprotein units i.e. α, β, γ, δ have been prepared from the electric organs of various species of *Torpedo* (Lindstrom *et al.*, 1979a). Antisera against whole ACR or to the subunits of this receptor have been prepared with a view to study the antigenic specificities of ACR (Lindstrom *et al.*, 1978, 1979b).

A real breakthrough in the fine analysis of antigenic specificities of ACR was carried out by Tzartos and Lindstrom (1980) who have obtained 17 hybridoma cell lines producing monoclonal antibodies against various antigenic determinants of electric organs of *Torpedo*. These monoclonal antibodies discriminate four categories of antigenic determinants. (1) antigenic determinants unique to each subunit of ACR of *Torpedo;* (2) antigenic determinants shared by α and β subunits; (3) antigenic determinants shared by γ and δ subunits; and (4) antigenic determinants which cross-reacted with ACR from other species.

Anti-ACR antibodies as well as the antibodies prepared from patients with myasthenia gravis cause the decrease of the number of ACR at the neuromuscular junction. This can be measured and quantitated by the binding of $[^{125}I]\alpha$-bungarotoxin, a purified snake toxin which binds specifically to ACR. Heineman *et al.* (1977) have shown that anti-ACR antibodies increased the rate of the degradation sixfold. The normal process of degradation of ACR is through the internalization and proteolysis by muscle. The binding of antibodies to ACR probably triggers and accelerates the degradation of receptor, since it was shown that the shedding of the complex of ^{125}I-labeled Bu-ACR was not increased significantly in the presence of antibodies (Stanley and Drachman, 1978). The increased degradation of ACR by antibodies leads to a decrease of sensitivity of cells to acetylcholine.

These few examples indicate that antibodies specific for the receptor of various somatic nonlymphoid cells for hormones or neurotransmitters can profoundly alter the function of these cells. In some circumstances the antibodies can mimic the functions of hormones and in others circumstances can accelerate and trigger the degradation of the receptors and, therefore, decrease the sensitivity of the cell for the transmitters.

In any event, a striking parallelism can be drawn between the effects of anti-receptor antibodies on somatic nonlymphoid cells and on the effects of anti-isotype, anti-allotype, and anti-idiotype antibodies on lymphocytes which can either stimulate or suppress the lymphocytic functions. The increase of [^{3}H]thymidine incorporation by anti-isotype, anti-allotype, and anti-Id antibodies as well as the priming of precursor of B cells and of helper T cells by anti-Id antibodies represent phenomena in which the antibodies clearly mimic the stimulating activity of antigen. Conversely, the isotype, allotype, and idiotype suppression induced by corresponding antibodies mimic the unresponsiveness of B and T lymphocytes caused by antigen.

II. Mimicry of Hormone and Vitamin Properties by Anti-Id Antibodies

Very provocative new findings suggest that anti-Id antibodies against the anti-insulin- or anti-retinol-binding protein antibodies mimic the effects of the binding of insulin- or retinol-binding protein to their corresponding cell receptors. These data indicate that a close resemblance could exist between the functional network of the immune system and of nonlymphoid somatic cells.

The sera of various mammalian species contain a protein which binds specifically vitamin A [retinol-binding protein (RBP)]. This RBP recognizes specifically a combining-site-like structure of serum prealbumin. In fact, the serum prealbumin binds RBP. RBP interacts specifically with the receptor associated with the membrane of various cells, such as the epithelial intestinal cells.

Sege and Peterson (1978a) have prepared in the rabbits anti-Id antibodies against rat anti-RBP. Rabbit antibodies were specific for Id determinants expressed on rat antibodies against RBP. The anti-Id antibodies, which strongly bind the rat anti-RBP antibodies, bind a very small amount of prealbumin. One milliliter of rabbit anti-Id serum bound 160 ng of human prealbumin and 120 ng of rat prealbumin. By contrast 1 ml of rabbit anti-rat prealbumin binds 150 μg of rat prealbumin and only 10 ng of human prealbumin. These results indicated that anti-Id antibodies have been directed against anti-RBP antibodies and not against prealbumin. In spite of their failure to interact with prealbumin, these anti-Id antibodies inhibited the binding of RBP to the RBP binding site of the prealbumin. This observation suggests a similarity between Id determinants of rat anti-RBP antibodies and the RBP binding site of prealbumin. The conclusion of this observation was supported by other two lines of evidence: (1) Anti-Id antibodies inhibited the binding of RBP to the receptor associated to the membrane of rat intestine epithelial cells. (2) Anti-Id antibodies prevented the uptake of labeled retinol by intestine cells, a process which is mediated by RBP.

A similar interaction was encountered in the insulin system. Sege and Peterson (1978b) have prepared in the rabbits anti-Id antibodies against rat anti-bovine insulin antibodies. The specificity of these anti-Id antibodies was carefully determined. The similarity between anti-Id antibodies and the binding site of insulin to the insulin receptor was supported by the results of two kinds of experiments.

In the first experimental system it was shown that anti-Id antibodies inhibited the binding of labeled-insulin to the insulin receptor of fat cells. This inhibition was specific since the inhibitory effect of anti-Id antibodies was removed by passing the anti-Id antibodies over a rat anti-insulin antibody adsorbant and was not affected by passing over a rat anti-RBP antibody adsorbant.

In addition it was shown that to some extent anti-Id antibodies can mimic some insulin properties, such as the increase of the uptake of α-aminobutyric by young rat thymocytes. The incubation of young rat thymocytes with 5 mg IgG fraction of rabbit anti-Id antibodies caused an increase of the uptake of $[^{14}C]\alpha$-aminobutyric comparable to that obtained with 5 μg insulin.

These findings indicate that anti-Id antibodies specific for Id determinants of rat anti-insulin or anti-RBP antibodies display some properties similar to those of the antigens (i.e., insulin and RBP) used for immunization. Furthermore, they are able to mimic some properties of the binding of insulin or RBP to cell surface receptor. Therefore, these results suggest that there is a similarity between anti-Id antibodies and the binding site of insulin or RBP to receptor and/or a similarity between Id determinants of anti-insulin and anti-RBP antibodies and the receptor site of the insulin and RBP receptors. Only the existence of such similarities could explain the mimicry of hormonal effects by anti-Id antibodies. These experiments provided the first evidence of homobodies (i.e., anti-Id antibodies as internal images of the antigen).

These observations have opened the way for future fruitful investigations of the possibility to monitor the autoimmune diseases in which the antibodies against the receptor play a well-established pathological role.

III. Autoimmune Anti-Receptor Diseases

The hypothesis of "immunopharmacological block" advanced by Lennon and Carnegie (1971) considered that some autoimmune diseases are due to anti-receptor antibodies which alter the accessibility of circulating hormones or neurotransmitters to their corresponding cell receptors. Several findings indicate that some autoimmune diseases are associated with anti-receptor antibodies.

A. Graves' Disease

Graves' disease is an autoimmune disorder in which the hyperthyroidism is associated with autoantibodies against the receptor of thyroid cells for thyroid-stimulating hormone (TSH).

Adams and Purves (1956, cited by Carnegie and Mackay 1975) found in the sera of these patients an immunoglobulin which stimulates human thyroid cells but not mouse thyroid cells. Later, several reports have shown that autoantibodies found in the sera of patients with Graves' disease inhibited the binding of TSH to thyroid membrane. McLachlan *et al.,* (1977) have succeeded in producing *in vitro* these autoantibodies by culturing the lymphocytes from patients with Graves' disease with PWM.

The anti-receptor properties of these autoantibodies were tested *in vitro* in two experimental systems. In the first system it was shown that IgG produced by PWM-stimulated lymphocytes from Graves' disease patients inhibited the binding of labeled TSH on thyroid membrane. The second system shows that these antibodies mimic the binding of TSH to TSH receptor by increasing the permeability of the lysosomes of thyroid cells. These results demonstrated clearly that autoantibodies were specific for the TSH receptor of thyroid cells.

B. Myasthenia Gravis

Most patients with myasthenia gravis have humoral antibodies against the acetylcholine receptor (ACR) of the motor end plate. The role of these autoantibodies in the pathogenesis of myasthenia gravis was substantiated by various experimental findings.

Experimental myasthenia gravis disease was induced in various mammalian species (rabbits, rats, guinea pigs, and monkeys) by immunization with purified ACR from the electric organs of various species of *Torpedo* and *Electrophorus* (Patrick and Lindstrom, 1973; Sugiyama *et al.*, 1973; Hazdai *et al.*, 1975; Lennon *et al.*, 1975; Lindstrom *et al.*, 1976).

The induction of antibodies against ACR of *Electrophorus,* which shares a cross-reactive antigen with the ACR of various mammalian species, resulted in an autoimmune myasthenia gravis syndrome. The animals enter a chronic phase of weakness which coincides with the occurrence of anti-ACR antibodies.

Claudio and Raftery (1980) have shown that only antibodies directed against the ACR and not against other contaminants are able to induce experimental autoimmune myasthenia gravis syndrome.

The skeletal muscle has two types of ACR: junctional and extrajunctional. Both receptors express a common antigen, and extrajunctional receptors bear an additional specific antigen. Weinberg and Hall (1979) have demonstrated that anti-ACR antibodies found in the sera of patients with myasthenia gravis are specific for the antigens of extrajunctional receptors. The autoanti-ACR antibodies from patients with myasthenia gravis-like anti-ACR antibodies induced by experimental immunization with purified receptors from various species of *Torpedo* or *Electrophorus* accelerate the degradation of ACR. Stanley and Drachman (1978) have found that the IgG fraction of sera from patients with myasthenia gravis accelerated the degradation of ACR either after administration *in vivo* into the mice or *in vitro* incubation with mouse muscle cells. This degradation was measured by both the loss of the ability to bind labeled α-bungarotoxin and by a decreased sensitivity to acetylcholine.

The breakdown of tolerance for ACR, which leads to the occurrence of autoanti-ACR antibodies, is linked to genetic factors. Thus, the *HLA-8* haplotype was frequently associated with myasthenia gravis in young women, whereas the *HLA-2* haplotype was associated with patients who have myasthenia gravis, thymoma, and myoid antibodies.

Studies in mice have shown that the occurrence of experimental myasthenia gravis autoimmune diseases can be under the control of *Ir* genes of MHC. The incidence of the disease and of anti-ACR antibodies was studied in various strains of mice immunized with 10 μg of purified *Torpedo california* ACR.

All the strains studied produced a high titer (7–10 ln units) of anti-ACR receptor. By contrast, while the mice of H-2 types a, b, d, and k developed clinical signs of weakness, the mice of H-2 types r and s did not (Fuchs *et al.*, 1976). These studies strongly indicate that anti-ACR antibodies which occur in myasthenia gravis and which induce an accelerated degradation of ACR play an inportant role in the dramatic decrease of the sensitivity to acetylcholine and therefore in the pathogenesis of this disease.

C. Diabetic Syndrome with Severe Insulin Resistance

Kahn *et al.* (1976) described a second subtype of acanthosis nigricans (type B syndrome) seen in old patients and characterized by a severe insulin resistance, hypergammaglobulinemia, proteinuria, leukopenia, alopecia, arthralgia, and enlarged salivary gland. The pathogenesis of the insulin resistance appeared clearly related to the inability of insulin to bind to its receptor. Field *et al.* (1961) already observed that insulin did not increase the uptake of glucose by fat cells of patients with an insulin-resistant diabetes compared with the fat cells from normal subjects or diabetic subjects sensitive to insulin. Kahn *et al.* (1976) associated the insulin resistance observed in the patients with type B syndrome to the presence of circulating anti-insulin receptor antibodies.

Flier *et al.* (1975) found that in six patients the binding of ^{125}I-labeled insulin to insulin receptors of human blood monocytes was only 5 to 30% of normal. The role of auto anti-receptor antibodies was demonstrated by the ability to compete with the binding of labeled insulin to the insulin receptor of four cell types: human peripheral blood monocytes, LM-9 lymphocyte line, avian erythrocytes, and rat liver plasma membrane. Cultured lymphocytes incubated with 1 : 2 diluted serum bound only 20% of insulin over the control, whereas the binding of growth hormone was not affected. From these findings it was concluded that autoantibody against the insulin receptor was responsible for the resistance to insulin observed in the case of these diabetic patients.

IV. Effects of Anti-Id Antibodies in Autoimmune Diseases

The breakdown of the tolerance against self-antigens leads to the appearance of autoantibodies which are responsible for the pathogenesis of various autoimmune diseases. These autoantibodies bear Id determinants, and in some cases they can express an IdX. Kunkel *et al.* (1974) have shown that human IgM myeloma protein which exhibited an autoreactivity for Fc fragment of human IgG can express an IdX.

The identification of IdX on anti-Id autoantibodies could open new ways for the manipulation of the autoimmune response and an eventual new therapeutic approach to autoimmune diseases.

Anti-Id antibodies against anti-ACR antibodies were prepared by Schwartz *et al.* (1978b) by immunization with syngeneic spleen cells educated with ACR. The rationale behind this method of preparation of anti-Id autoantibodies was that the anti-ACR antibody response is dependent on T cell help, and therefore helper T cells should bear on their receptors the Id determinants of anti-ACR antibodies. Anti-Id antibodies were elicited in C57BL/6 mice by repeated intradermal immunizations with 5×10^7 ACR educated C57BL/6 spleen cells. The anti-idiotypic sera obtained by this method did not contain any appreciable amount of anti-ACR activity, and only Ig molecules of one distinct antibody specificity (i.e. for ACR) were recognized by anti-Id serum. Interestingly, the anti-Id antibodies interacted not only with C57BL/6 anti-ACR antibodies but also with anti-ACR antibodies produced by various strains of mice independently of their Igh-C (e.g., Ig-1[b], Ig-1[d], Ig-1[e], Ig-1[c] and Ig-1[a]) as well as with rabbit, rat, and monkey anti-ACR antibodies. It appears, therefore, that anti-ACR antibodies expressed an interspecies IdX which can be expected in the case of an evolutionary highly conserved antigen such as ACR.

Other examples of IdX on auto antibodies were provided by studies of spontaneous autoimmune thyroiditis in the BUF strain of rats. The occurrence of this disease is associated with anti-thyroglobulin antibodies. Zanetti and Bigazzi (1980) prepared in the rabbit an anti-Id antiserum against BUF rat auto anti-thyroglobulin antibodies. This anti-Id serum interacted with autoantibodies from another 15 rats with spontaneous autoimmune disorder. These results indicated that anti-thyroglobulin autoantibodies from BUF rats possess a similar or an IdX.

The utilization of anti-Id antibodies for treating and managing an autoimmune disease was performed by Brown *et al.* (1979) in the case of autoimmune tubule interstitial nephritis in guinea pigs. Strain 13 guinea pigs immunized with rabbit tubular basement membrane developed a severe tubulointerstitial nephritis associated with autoantibodies. These autoantibodies eluted from kidney of guinea pigs with autoimmune disease were used as immunogen in order to prepare in the rabbits anti-Id antibodies.

This anti-Id serum was administered to guinea pigs before the immunization with tubular basement membrane antigen. Animals which received the anti-Id antibodies had significantly less disease and a lower titer of autoantibodies. These results indicate that anti-Id antibodies inhibited the development of tubulointerstitial nephritis in guinea pigs. Therefore, these results suggest that anti-Id antibodies can be used to prevent the development of an experimental autoimmune disease.

In summary, these findings indicate that the immune network regulatory mechanisms of immune apparatus is a more general mechanism which regulates the functions of nonlymphoid cells and which can have important implications in the pathogenesis of various diseases. Furthermore, anti-idiotype antibodies can be used in certain situations to manage the development of autoimmune diseases.

References

Aasted, B., Sogn, J. A., and Kindt, T. J. (1976). *J. Immunol.* **116**, 387.

Abdou, N. I., and Abdou, N. L. (1975). *Ann. Intern. Med.* **83**, 42.

Adorni, L., Harvey, M., and Sercaz, E. E. (1979). *Eur. J. Immunol.* **9**, 906.

Aguet, M., Andersson, L. C., Andersson, R., Wight, E., Binz, H., and Wigzell, H. (1978). *J. Exp. Med.* **147**, 50.

Alevy, Y. G., and Bellone, C. J. (1979). *Fed. Proc., Fed. Am. Soc. Exp. Biol.* **38**, 1357.

Alevy, Y. G., and Bellone, C. J. (1980). *J. Exp. Med.* **151**, 528.

Alevy, Y. G., Witherspoon, C. D., Prange, C. A., and Bellone, C. J. (1980). *J. Immunol.* **124**, 217.

Amerding, D., and Katz, D. (1975). *J. Exp. Med.* **140**, 19.

Andersson, L. C., Aguet, M., Wight, E., Andersson, R., Binz, H , and Wigzell, H. (1977). *J. Exp. Med.* **146**, 1124.

Archer, O. K., Sutherland, D. E. R., and Good, R. A. (1964). *Lab. Invest.* **13**, 259.

Augustin, A., and Cosenza, H. (1976). *Eur. J. Immunol.* **6**, 497.

Bach, B. A., Green, M. I., Benacerraf, B., and Nisonoff, A. (1979). *J. Exp. Med.* **149**, 1084.

Bankert, R. B., and Pressman, D. (1976). *J. Immunol.* **117**, 457.

Belgrau, D., and Wilson, D. B. (1978). *J. Exp. Med.* **148**, 103.

Belgrau, D., and Wilson, D. B. (1979). *J. Exp. Med.* **149**, 234.

Benacerraf, B., and Dorf, M. E. (1977). *Eur. J. Immunol.* **7**, 865.

Benacerraf, B., and McDevitt, H. O. (1972). *Science* **175**, 273.

Berek, C., Taylor, B. A., and Eichmann, (1978). *J. Exp. Med.* **149**, 1164.

Binz, H., and Lindemann J. (1972). *J. Exp. Med.* **136**, 872.

Binz, H., and Wigzell, H. (1975a). *J. Exp. Med.* **142**, 197.

Binz, H., and Wigzell, H. (1975b). *J. Exp. Med.* **142**, 1218.

Binz, H., and Wigzell, H. (1975c). *J. Exp. Med.* **142**, 1231.

Binz, H., and Wigzell, H. (1975d). *J. Scand. Immunol.* 4, 531.

Binz, H., and Wigzell, H. (1976). *Scand. J. Immunol.* 5, 553.

Binz, H., and Wigzell, H. (1978). *J. Exp. Med.* 147, 63.

Binz, H., Lindemann, J., and Wigzell, H. (1974). *J. Exp. Med.* 140, 731.

Binz, H., Wigzell, H., and Bazin, H. (1976). *Nature (London)* 264, 639.

Binz, H., Frischknecht, H., Shen, F. W., and Wigzell, H. (1979a). *J. Exp. Med.* 149, 940.

Binz, H., Frischknecht, H., Mercolli, C., Dunst, S., and Wigzell, H. (1979b). *J. Exp. Med.* 149, 1084.

Binz, H., Frischknecht, H., and Wigzell, H. (1979c). *Ann. Immunol. (Paris)* 130C, 273.

Black, S. J., Hammerling, G. J., Rajewsky, K., and Eichmann, K. (1976). *J. Exp. Med.* 143, 846.

Bona, C. (1979a). *In* "Cell Biology and Immunology of Leukocyte Function" (M. Quastel, ed.), p. 769. Academic Press, New York.

Bona, C. (1979b). *Prog. Allergy* 26, 97.

Bona, C. (1979c). *In* "The Molecular Basis of Immune Cell Function" (J. G. Kaplan, ed.) p. 161. Elsevier-North Holland Biomed. Press, Amsterdam.

Bona, C. (1980a). *In* "Progress in Myeloma" (M. Potter, ed.), p. 209. Elsevier-North Holland, New York.

Bona, C. (1980b). *In* "Membrane Receptors and Immune Response" (E. Cohen, H. Kohler, and D. Rowley, eds.), p. 263. Alan R. Liss, Inc., New York.

Bona, C. (1981a). *In* "Lymphocytic Regulation by Antibodies" (C. Bona and P. A. Cazenave, eds.). Wiley, New York (in press).

Bona, C. (1981b). *In* "B Lymphocytes in the Immune Response" (N. Klinman, D. Mosier, I. Scher, and E. Vitetta, eds.), p. 437. Elsevier-North Holland, New York.

Bona, C., and Cazenave, P. A. (1977). *J. Exp. Med.* 146, 881.

Bona, C., and Cazenave, P. A. (1981). *In* "Lymphocyte Regulation by Antibodies" (C. Bona and P. A. Cazenave, eds.). Wiley, New York.

Bona, C., and Fauci, A. (1980). *J. Clin. Invest.* 65, 761.

Bona, C., and Hiernaux, J. (1981). *Crit. Rev. Immunol.* (in press).

Bona, C., and Paul, W. E. (1979a). *J. Exp. Med.* 149, 542.

Bona, C., and Paul, W. E. (1979b). *In* "Cells of Immunoglobulin Synthesis" (B. Pernis and H. Vogel, eds.), p. 291. Academic Press, New York.

Bona, C., Audibert, F., Juy, D., and Chédid, L. (1976). *Clin. Exp. Immunol.* 26, 258.

Bona, C., Dubiski, S., and Cinader, B. (1977). *Ann Immunol. (Paris)* 128C, 38.

Bona, C., Lieberman, R., Chien, C. C., Moud, J., House, S., Green, I., and Paul, W. E. (1978). *J. Immunol.* 120, 1436.

Bona, C., Cazenave, P. A., and Paul, W. E. (1979a). *Ann. Immunol. (Paris)* 130C, 303.

Bona, C., Stein, K. E., Lieberman, R., and Paul, W. E. (1979b). *Immunology* 16, 1093.

Bona, C., Lieberman, R., House, S., Green, I., and Paul, W. E. (1979c). *J. Immunol.* 122, 1614.

Bona, C., Mond, J., Stein, S., Lieberman, R., and Paul, W. E. (1979d). *J. Immunol.* 123, 1484.

Bona, C., Hooghe, R., Cazenave, P. A., Le Guern, C., and Paul, W. E. (1979c). *J. Exp. Med.* 149, 815.

Bona, C., Mond, J. J., and Paul, W. E. (1980a). *J. Exp. Med.* 151, 224.

Bona, C., Mongini, P. K. A., Stein, K. G., and Paul, W. E. (1980b). *J. Exp. Med.* 151, 1334.

Bona, C., Heber-Katz, E., and Paul, W. E. (1981). *J. Exp. Med.* **153**, 951.

Bordenave, G. R. (1975). *Immunology* **28**, 635.

Bossing-Schneider, R. (1979). *Immunology* **36**, 527.

Bottomly, K., and Mosier, D. E. (1979). *J. Exp. Med.* **150**, 1399.

Bottomly, K., Mathieson, B. J., and Mosier, D. E. (1978). *J. Exp. Med.* **148**, 915.

Bottomly, K., Janneway, C. A., Mathieson, B. J., and Mosier, D. E. (1980). *Eur. J. Immunol.* **10**, 159.

Brandt, D. C., and Jaton, J. C. (1978). *J. Immunol.* **121**, 1188.

Braun, M., and Saal, F. (1977). *Cell. Immunol.* **30**, 254.

Brent, B. W., and Nisonoff, A. (1970). *J. Exp. Med.* **132**, 951.

Briles, D. E., and Davie, J. M. (1980). *J. Exp. Med.* **152**, 151.

Briles, D. E., and Krause, R. M. (1974). *J. Immunol.* **113**, 522.

Brown, C. A., Carey, K., and Colvin, R. B. (1979). *J. Immunol.* **123**, 2102.

Brown, J. C., and Rodkey, L. S. (1979). *J. Exp. Med.* **150**, 67.

Burnet, F. M. (1959). "The Clonal Selection Theory of Acquired Immunity." Cambridge Univ. Press, Oxford.

Buttin, G., Juy, D., Medrano, L., Legrain, P., LeGuern, C., and Cazenave, P. A. (1979). *In* "The Molecular Basis of Immune Cell Function" (J. E. Kaplan, ed.), p. 331. Elsevier-North Holland Biomed. Press, Amsterdam.

Cancro, M.P., Sigal, N. H., and Klinman, N. R. (1977). *J. Exp. Med.* **147**, 1.

Capra, J. D., and Kehoe, J. M. (1974). *Proc. Natl. Acad Sci. U.S.A.* **71**, 4032.

Capra, J. D., Kehoe, J. M., Williams, R. C., Feizi, T., and Kunkel, H. G. (1972). *Proc. Natl. Acad Sci. U.S.A.* **69**, 40.

Capra, J. D., Tung, A. S., and Nisonoff, A. (1977). *J. Immunol.* **119**, 993.

Carnegie, P. R., and Mackay, I. R. (1975). *Lancet* **1**, 684.

Carson, D., and Weigert, M. (1973). *Proc. Natl. Acad. Sci. U.S.A.* **70**, 235.

Cavaillon, J. M., Bona, C., Cazenave, P. A., and Cinader, B. (1977). *J. Methods Immunol.* **14**, 355.

Cazenave, P. A. (1977). *Proc. Natl. Acad. Sci. U.S.A.* **74**, 5122.

Cazenave, P. A., and Oudin, J. (1973). *C. R. Hebd. Seances Acad. Sci.* **276**, 243.

Cazenave, P. A., Ternynck, T., and Avrameas, A. (1974). *Proc. Natl. Acad. Sci. U.S.A.* **71**, 4500.

Cazenave, P. A., Cavaillon, J. M., and Bona, C. (1977a). *Immunol. Rev.* **34**, 34.

Cazenave, P. A., Juy, D., and Bona, C. (1977b). *In* "Developmental Immunobiology" (J. B. Solomon and J. D. Horton, eds.), p. 347. Elsevier-North Holland, New York.

Cazenave, P. A., Juy, D., and Bona, C. (1978). *J. Immunol.* **120**, 444.

Cazenave, P. A., Le Guern, C., Bona, C., and Buttin, G. (1980). *In* "Membrane Receptors and the Immune Response" (E. Cohen, H. Kohler, and D. Rowley, eds.), p. 359. Alan R. Liss, Inc., New York.

Claflin, J. L., and Cubberley, M. (1978). *J. Immunol.* **121**, 1410.

Claflin, J. L., and Davie J. M. (1974). *J. Immunol.* **114**, 1678.

Claflin, J. L., and Davie, J. M. (1975a). *J. Immunol.* **114**, 70.

Claflin, J. L., and Davie, J. M. (1975b). *J. Exp. Med.* **141**, 1073.

Claflin, J. L., and Rudikoff, S. (1979). *J. Immunol.* **122**, 1402.

Claflin, J. L., Lieberman, R., and Davie, J. M. (1974). *J. Exp. Med.* **139**, 58.

Claudio, T. R., and Raftery, M. A. (1980). *J. Immunol.* **124**, 1130.

Clevinger, B., Schilling, J., Hood, L., and Davie, J. M. (1980). *J. Exp. Med.* **151**, 1059.

Cohn, M. (1971). *Cell. Immunol.* 1, 461.

Coombs, R. R. A., Gurner, B. W., Janneway, C. A., Wilson, A. B., Gell, P. G. H., and Kelus, A. S. (1970a). *Immunology* 18, 417.

Coombs, R. R. A., Gurner, B. A., McConnell, I., and Munro, A. (1970b). *Int. Arch. Allergy Appl. Immunol.* 39, 280.

Cooper, M. D., and Lawton, A. R. (1979). *In* "Cells of Immunoglobulin Synthesis" (B. Pernis and H. J. Vogel, eds.), p. 411. Academic Press, New York.

Cooper, M., Kubagawa, H., Vogler, L. B., Levitt, D., and Lawton, A. R. (1979). *In* "B Lymphocytes in the Immune Response (M. Cooper, D. E. Mosier, I. Scher, and E. S. Vitetta, eds.), p. 181. Elsevier-North Holland, New York.

Cosenza, H. (1976). *Eur. J. Immunol.* 6, 114.

Cosenza, H., and Kohler, H. (1972). *Proc. Natl. Acad. Sci. U.S.A.* 69, 2701.

Cosenza, H., Julius, M. H., and Augustin, A. (1977). *Immunol. Rev.* 34, 3.

Coutinho, A., Forni, L., and Blomberg, B. (1978). *J. Exp. Med.* 148, 862.

Cramer, M., Krawinkel, U., Melchlers, I., Imanishi-Kari, T., Ben-Neriah, Y., Givol, D., and Rajewski, K. (1979). *Eur. J. Immunol.* 9, 332.

Crone, M., Koch, C., and Simonsen, M. (1972). *Transplant. Rev.* 10, 36.

Daley, J. M., Gebel, H. M., and Lynch, R. (1978). *J. Immunol.* 120, 1620.

de Saint Martin, J., Mukoyama, H., and Eyquem, A. (1978). *C. R. Hebd. Seances Acad. Sci.* 281, 1185.

Dohi, Y., and Nisonoff, A. (1973). *J. Exp. Med.* 150, 909.

DuClos, T., and Kim, B. S. (1977). *J. Immunol.* 119, 1769.

Eichmann, K. (1974). *Eur. J. Immunol.* 4, 236.

Eichmann, K. (1975a). *Eur. J. Immunol.* 5, 511.

Eichmann, K. (1975b). *Immunogenetics* 2, 491.

Eichmann, K. (1978). *Adv. Immunol.* 26, 195.

Eichmann, K., and Berek, C. (1973). *Eur. J. Immunol.* 3, 559.

Eichmann, K., and Kindt, T. J. (1974). *J. Exp. Med.* 134, 532.

Eichmann, K., and Rajewsky, K. (1975). *Eur. J. Immunol.* 5, 661.

Eichmann, K., Couthino, A., and Melchers, F. (1977). *J. Exp. Med.* 146, 1436.

Eichmann, K., Falk, I., and Rajewsky, K. (1978). *J. Eur. Immunol.* 8, 853.

Eig, B. M., Ju, S. -T., and Nisonoff, A. (1977). *J. Exp. Med.* 146, 1574.

Eisen, H. N., Sakato, N., and Hall, S. J. (1975). *Transplant. Proc.* 7, 209.

Eyquem, A., and Bona, C. (1977). *Clin. Immunol. Immunopathol.* 7, 1.

Fathman, C. G., Pisetsky, D. S., and Sachs, D. H. (1977). *J. Exp. Med.* 145, 569.

Feldman, M., (1972). *J. Exp. Med.* 136, 737.

Feldman, M., and Basten, A. (1972). *J. Exp. Med.* 136, 722.

Fernandez, C., and Moller, G. (1978). *J. Exp. Med.* 147, 645.

Fernandez, C., and Moller, G. (1979). *Proc. Natl. Acad. Sci. U.S.A.* 76, 5944.

Fernandez, C., Hammarström, L., Moller, G., Primi, D., and Smith, C. J. E. (1979). *Immunol. Rev.* 43, 3.

Field, J. B., Johnson, P., and Herring, B. (1961). *J. Clin. Invest.* 40, 1672.

Flier, J. S., Kahn, R., Roth, J., and Bar, R. S. (1975). *Science* 188, 63.

Forni, L., Cazenave, P. A., Cosenza, H., Forsbeck, K., and Coutinho, A. (1979). *Nature (London)* 280, 241.

Freedman, P., Autry, J. R., Tokuda, S., and Williams, R. C. (1976). *J. Natl. Cancer Inst.* 56, 735.

Fu, S. M., Winchester, R. J., Reizi, T., Walzer, P. D., and Kunkel, H. G. (1974a). *Proc. Natl. Acad. Sci. U.S.A.* 71, 4487.

Fu, S. M., Winchester, R. J., and Kunkel, H. G. (1974b). *J. Exp. Med.* **139**, 451.

Fu, S. M., Winchester, R. J., and Kunkel, H. G. (1974c). *J. Immunol.* **114**, 250.

Fu, S. M., Winchester, J., and Kunkel, H. G. (1975). *J. Immunol.* **114**, 250.

Fuchs, S., Nevo, D., and Tarrab-Hazdai, R. (1976). *Nature (London)* **263**, 329.

Fung, J. J., Gelson, K., Ward, R., and Kohler, H. (1980). *In* "Membrane, Receptors and the Immune Response" (E. P. Cohen and H. Kohler, Eds.), p. 203. Alan R. Liss, New York.

Gathings, W. E., Lawton, A. R., and Cooper, M. D. (1977). *Eur. J. Immunol.* **7**, 804.

Geckler, W. R., Blumberg, B., dePreval, C., and Cohn, M. (1977). *Cold Spring Harbor Symp. Quant. Biol.* **41**, 165.

Geczy, A. F., Geczy, C. L., and de Weck, A. L. (1976). *J. Exp. Med.* **144**, 226.

Geha, R. S. (1977). *J. Exp. Med.* **145**, 1436.

Geha, R. S., Mudawwar, F., and Schneeberger, E. (1977). *J. Exp. Med.* **145**, 1436.

Gerhart, P. J., and Cebra, J. J. (1979). *J. Exp. Med.* **149**, 216.

Germain, R. N., Ju, S. T., Kipps, T. J., Benacerraf, B., and Dorf, M. E. (1979). *J. Exp. Med.* **149**, 613.

Gilman-Sachs, A., Dray, S., and Horng, W. J. (1980). *J. Immunol.* **125**, 96.

Goidl, E. A., Schrater, A. F., Siskind, G. F., and Thorbeck, G. J. (1979). *J. Exp. Med.* **150**; 154.

Granato, D., Braun, D. G., and Vassalli, P. (1974). *J. Immunol.* **113**, 417.

Grey, H. M., Mannik, M., and Kunkel, H. G. (1965). *J. Exp. Med.* **121**, 561.

Haimovich, J., Eisen, H. N., Hurvitz, E., and Givol, D. (1972). *Biochemistry* **11**, 2389.

Haines, A. K., Siskind, G. W. (1980). *J. Immunol.* **124**, 1878.

Hamers-Casterman, C., and Hamers, R. (1975). *Immunogenetics* **1**, 598.

Hammerling, G., and Eichmann, K. (1976). *Eur. J. Immunol.* **6**, 565.

Hansburg, D., Briles, D. E., and Davie, J. M. (1976). *J. Immunol.* **117**, 563.

Hansburg, D., Briels, D. E., and Davie, J. M. (1977). *J. Immunol.* **119**, 1406.

Hardy, B., Globerson, A., and Danon, D. (1973). *Cell. Immunol.* **9**, 282.

Hart, D. A., Wang, A. L., Pawlak, L. L., and Nisonoff, A. (1972). *J. Exp. Med.* **135**, 1293.

Harvey, M. A., Adorni, L., Miller, A., and Sercaz, E. (1979). *Nature (London)* **281**, 594.

Haughton, G., Lanier, L., Babcock, G. F., and Lynes, M. A. (1978). *J. Immunol.* **121**, 2358.

Hayward, A. R., Simons, M. A., Lawton, A. R., Mage, R. G., and Cooper, M. D. (1978). *J. Exp. Med.* **148**, 1367.

Hazdai, R., Aharanov, A., Silman, I., Fuchs, S., and Abramsky, O. (1975). *Nature (London)* **256**, 128.

Heinemann, S., Bevan, S., Kullberg, R., Lindstrom, J., and Rice, J. (1977). *Proc. Natl. Acad. Sci. U.S.A.* **74**, 3090.

Helman, M., Shreier, I., and Givol, D. (1976). *J. Immunol.* **117**, 1933.

Hetzelberger, D., and Eichmann, K. (1978a). *Eur. J. Immunol.* **8**, 833.

Hetzelberger, D., and Eichmann, K. (1978b). *Eur. J. Immunol.* **8**, 846.

Hiernaux, J. (1977). *Immunochemistry* **14**, 733.

Hiernaux, J., and Bona, C. (1981). *In* "Lymphocytic Regulation by Antibodies" (C. Bona and P. A. Cazenave, eds.), p. 269. Wiley, New York.

Hiernaux, J., Bona, C., and Baker, P. A. (1981). *J. Exp. Med.* **153**, 1004.

Hilschmann, N., and Craig, L. C. (1965). *Proc. Natl. Acad. Sci. U.S.A.* **53**, 1403.

Hoffmann, G. W. (1975). *Eur. J. Immunol.* **5**, 638.

Holm, G., Melsted, H., Petterson, D., and Biberfield, P. (1977). *Immunol. Rev.* **34**, 139.

Hopper, J. E., and Nisonoff, A. (1971). *Adv. Immunol.* **13**, 57.

Horng, W. J., Gilman-Sachs, A., and Dray, S. (1981). *In* "Lymphocytic Regulation by Antibodies" (C. Bona and P. A. Cazenave, eds.) p. 139. Wiley, New York.

Howard, J. G., and Hale, C. (1976). *Eur. J. Immunol.* **6**, 486.

Hunter, P., and Kettman, J. R. (1974). *Proc. Natl. Acad. Sci. U.S.A.* **71**, 512.

Hurley, J. H., Fu, S. M., Kunkel, H. G., McKenna, G., and Scharff, M. D. (1978). *Proc. Natl. Acad Sci. U.S.A.* **75**, 5706.

Hurme, M., Karjalainen, K., and Mäkelä, O. (1980). *Scand. J. Immunol.* **11**, 241.

Imanish, T., and Mäkelä, O. (1973). *Eur. J. Immunol.* **3**, 323.

Imanishi, T., Hurme, M., Serves, H., and Mäkelä, O. (1975). *Eur. J. Immunol.* **5**, 198.

Jack, R. S., Imanishi, K., and Rajewsky, K. (1977). *Eur. J. Immunol.* **8**, 554.

Jackson, S., and Mestecky, J. (1979). *J. Exp. Med.* **150**, 1265.

Jacobs, S., Chang, K. J., and Cuatrecasas, P. (1978). *Science* **200**, 1283.

Janneway, C. A. (1975). *J. Immunol.* **114**, 1394.

Janneway, C. A., and Paul, W. E. (1973). *Eur. J. Immunol.* **3**, 340.

Janneway, C. A., and Paul, W. E. (1976). *J. Exp. Med.* **144**, 1641.

Janneway, C. A., Murgita, R. A., Weinbaum, F. L., Asofsky, R., and Wigzell, H., (1977). *Proc. Natl. Acad. Sci. U.S.A.* **74**, 4582.

Jerne, N. K. (1976). p. 93. Academic Press, New York.

Jerne, N. K. (1974). *Ann. Immunol. (Paris)* **125C**, 373.

Jorgensen, T., and Hannestad, K. (1979). *Scand. J. Immunol.* **8**, 635.

Jorgensen, T., Gaudernack, G., and Hannestad, K. (1977). *Scand. J. Immunol.* **6**, 311.

Ju, S.-T., and Dorf, M. E. (1979). *Eur. J. Immunol.* **9**, 553.

Ju, S.-T., Gray, A., and Nisonoff, A. (1977). *J. Exp. Med.* **145**, 540.

Ju, S.-T., Kipps, T. J., Thèze, J., Benacerraf, B., and Dorf, M. E. (1978a). *J. Immunol.* **121**, 1034.

Ju, S.-T., Benacerraf, B., and Dorf, M. E. (1978b). *Proc. Natl. Acad. Sci. U.S.A.* **75**, 6192.

Ju, S.-T., Pierres, M., Waltenbaugh, C., Germain, R. N., Benacerraf, B., and Dorf, M. E. (1979a). *Proc. Natl. Acad. Sci. U.S.A.* **76**, 2942.

Ju, S.-T., Pierres, M., Germain, R. N., Benacerraf, B., and Dorf, M. (1979b). *J. Immunol.* **123**, 2505.

Ju, S.-T., Benacerraf, B., and Dorf, M. E. (1980). *J. Exp. Med.* **152**, 170.

Julin, M., Karajalainen, K., and Mäkelä, O. (1976). *Ann. Immunol. (Paris)* **127C**, 409.

Julius, M. H., and Hertzenberg, L. A. (1974). *J. Exp. Med.* **122**, 853.

Julius, M. H., Augustin, A. A., and Cosenza, H. (1977). *Nature (London)* **265**, 251.

Julius, M. H., Augustin, A. A., and Cosenza, H. (1978a). *In* "The Immune System: Genetics and Regulation" (E. Sercaz, L. A. Hertzenberg, and C. F. Fox, eds.), p. 179. Academic Press, New York.

Julius, M. H., Cosenza, H., and Augustin, A. A. (1978b). *Eur. J. Immunol.* **8**, 484.

Kabat, E. A. (1976). *Ann. Immunol. (Paris)* **127C**, 239.

Kabat, E. A., Wu, T. T., and Bilofsky, H. (1979). US Health Serv., Natl. Inst. Health, Washington, D.C.

Kahn, C. R., Flier, J. S., Bar, R. S., Archer, J. A., Gordon, P., Martin, M. M., and Roth, J. (1976). *N. Engl. J. Med.* **234**, 739.

Kaplan, R., and Quintanas, J. (1979a). *J. Exp. Med.* **149**, 267.

Kaplan, R. B., and Quintanas, J. (1979b). *J. Supramolec. Struct. suppl.* **3**, 266.

Karol, B. R., Reichlin, M., and Noble, R. W. (1977). *J. Exp. Med.* **146**, 435.

Karol, B. R., Rechlin, M., and Noble, R. W. (1978). *J. Exp. Med.* 148, 1488.

Katz, D. H., Greaves, M., Dorf, M. E., Dimuzio, H., and Benacerraf, B. (1975). *J. Exp. Med.* 141, 263.

Katz, S. I., Parker, D., and Turk, J. L. (1974). *Nature (London)* 251, 559.

Kelsoe, G., and Cerny, J. (1979). *Nature (London)* 279, 333.

Kelsoe, G., Isaak, D., and Cerny, J. (1980). *J. Exp. Med.* 151, 289.

Kim, B. S. (1979). *J. Exp. Med.* 149, 1371.

Kishimoto, T. (1979). *In* "B Lymphocytes in the Immune Response" (M. Cooper, D. Mosier, I. Scher, and E. S. Vitetta, eds.), p. 285. Elsevier-North Holland, New York.

Klaus, G. G. B. (1978). *Nature (London)* 272, 265.

Klinman, N. R. (1972). *J. Exp. Med.* 136, 241.

Klinman, N. R., Pickarol, A. R., Signal, N. H., Gerhart, P. J., Metcalf, E. S., and Pierce, S. K. (1976). *Ann. Immunol. (Paris)* 127C, 489.

Kluskens, L., and Kohler, H. (1974). *Proc. Natl. Acad. Sci. U.S.A.* 71, 5083.

Kohler, H. (1975). *Transplant. Rev.* 27, 24.

Kohler, H., Streyer, D. S., and Kaplan, D. R. (1974). *Science* 186, 643.

Kohler, H., Richardson, B. C., and Smyk, S. (1978). *J. Immunol.* 126, 233.

Kohler, H., Richardson, B. C., Rowley, D. A., and Smyk, S. (1977). *J. Immunol.* 119, 1979.

Koshland, M. E. (1967). *Cold Spring Harbor Symp. Quant. Biol.* 32, 119.

Krammer, P. H. (1978). *J. Exp. Med.* 147, 25.

Krammer, P. H., and Eichmann, K. (1977). *Nature (London)* 270, 733.

Krawinkel, W., Cramer, M., Mage, R. G., Kelus, A. S., and Rajewsky, K. (1977). *J. Exp. Med.* 146, 792.

Krawinkel, W., Cramer, M., Melchers, I., Imanishi-Kari, T., and Rajewsky, K. (1978). *J. Exp. Med.* 147, 1341.

Kubagawa, H., Vogler, L. B., Capra, J. D., Conrad, M. G., Lawton, A. R., and Cooper, M. D. (1979). *J. Exp. Med.* 150, 782.

Kubagawa, H., Vogler, L. B., Lawton, A. R., and Cooper, M. D. (1980). *In* "Progress in Myeloma" (M. Potter, ed.), p. 195. Elsevier-North Holland, New York.

Kunkel, H. G. (1970). *Fed. Proc., Fed. Am. Soc. Exp. Biol.* 9, 55.

Kunkel, H. G., Mannik, M., and Williams, R. C. (1963). *Science* 140, 1218.

Kunkel, H. G., Aguello, V., Joslin, F. G., Winchester, R. J., and Capra, J. D. (1973). *J. Exp. Med.* 137, 331.

Kunkel, H. G., Winchester, R. J., Joslin, F., and Capra, J. B. (1974). *J. Exp. Med.* 149, 128.

Kunkel, H. G., Joslin, F., and Hurley, J. (1976). *J. Immunol.* 116, 1532.

Lea, T., Førre, O. T., Michaelsen, T. E., and Natvig, J. B. (1979). *J. Immunol.* 122, 2413.

Lederberg, J. (1953). *Science* 129, 1643.

Lederberg, J. (1959). *Science (Washington, D.C.)* 129, 1649.

LeGuern, C., Ben Aissa, F., Juy, D., Mariame, B., Buttin, G., and Cazenave, P. A. (1974). *Ann. Immunol. (Paris)* 130C, 293.

Lennon, V. A., and Carnegie, P. K. (1971). *Lancet* 6, 630.

Lennon, V. A., Lindstrom, J. M., and Seybold, M. E. (1975). *J. Exp. Med.* 141, 1365.

Lewis, G. K., and Goodman, J. W. (1978). *J. Exp. Med.* 148, 915.

Lieberman, R., and Humphrey, W. (1971). *Proc. Natl. Acad. Sci. U.S.A.* 68, 2510.

Lieberman, R., and Humphrey, W. (1972). *J. Exp. Med.* 136, 1222.

Lieberman, R., Potter, M., Mushinski, E. B., Humphrey, W., and Rudikoff, S. (1974). *J. Exp. Med.* **139**, 983.

Lieberman, R., Potter, M., Humphrey, W., Jr., Mushinski, E. B., and Vrana, M. (1975). *J. Exp. Med.* **142**, 106.

Lieberman, R., Potter, M., Humphrey, W., and Chien, C. C. (1976). *J. Immunol.* **117**, 2105.

Lieberman, R., Vrana, M., Humphrey, W., Chien, C. C., and Potter, M. (1977). *J. Exp. Med.* **146**, 1294.

Lieberman, R., Bona, C., Chien, C. C., Stein, K. E., and Paul, W. E. (1979). *Ann. Immunol. (Paris)* **130C**, 247.

Lindemann, J. (1979). *Ann. Immunol. (Paris)* **130C**, 311.

Lindstrom, F. D., Hardy, W. R., Eberle, B. J., and Williams, R. C. (1973). *Ann. Intern. Med.* **78**, 837.

Lindstrom, J. M., Lennon, V. A., Seybold, M. E., and Whittingham, S. (1976). *Ann. N.Y. Acad. Sci.* **274**, 254.

Lindstrom, J., Einarson, B., and Merlie, J. (1978). *Proc. Natl. Acad. Sci. U.S.A.* **75**, 769.

Lindstrom, J. M., Merlie, J., and Yogeesnaran, G. (1979a). *Biochemistry* **18**, 4465.

Lindstrom, J. M., Walter (Nave) B., and Einarson, B. (1979b). *Biochemistry* **18**, 4470.

Lisowska-Bernstein, B., Rinwy, A., and Vassalli, P. (1973). *Proc. Natl. Acad. Sci. U.S.A.* **70**, 2879.

Lonai, P., Ben-Neriah, Y., Steinman, L., and Givol, D. (1978). *Eur. J. Immunol.* **8**, 827.

Lozner, E. C., Sachs, D. H., and Shearer, G. M. (1974). *J. Exp. Med.* **139**, 1204.

Lynch, R. G., Graft, R. J., Sirisinha, S., Simms, S. G., and Eisen, H. N. (1972). *Proc. Natl. Acad. Sci. U.S.A.* **69**, 1540.

Lynch, R. G., Rohrer, J. W., Odermatt, B., Gebel, H. M., Autry, J. R., and Hoover, R. G. (1979). *Immunol. Rev.* **48**, 47.

McConnell, I., Lachmann, P. J., and Givol, D. (1976). *Immunology* **30**, 841.

MacDonald, A. B., and Nisonoff, A. (1970). *J. Exp. Med.* **131**, 583.

McKearn, T. J., Stuart, F. P., and Fitch, F. W. (1974). *J. Immunol.* **113**, 1876.

McLachlan, S. M., Rees Smith, B., Petersen, W. B., Davies, T. F., and Hall, R. (1977). *Nature (London)* **270**, 447.

McMichel, A., Philips, J. M., Williamson, A. R., and Mäkelä, O. (1975). *Immunogenetics (N.Y.)* **2**, 161.

Mäkelä, O. (1970). *J. Analt. Rev.* **5**, 3.

Mäkelä, O., and Imanishi, T. (1975). *Eur. J. Immunol.* **5**, 202.

Mäkelä, O., and Karjalainen, K. (1977a). *Cold Spring Harbor Symp. Quant. Biol.* **118**, 41, 2161.

Mäkelä, O., and Karjalainen, K. (1977b). *Immunol. Rev.* **34**, 119.

Mäkelä, O., Karjalainen, K., Ju, S.-T., and Nisonoff, A. (1977). *Eur. J. Immunol.* **7**, 831.

Meinke, G. C., McConahey, P. J., and Spiegelberg, H. L. (1974). *Fed. Proc., Fed. Am. Soc. Exp. Biol.* **33**, 792.

Melchers, F., Andersson, J., and Phillips, R. A. (1977). *Cold Spring Harbor Symp. Quant. Biol.* **41**, 147.

Mellstadt, H. S., Hammerström, S., and Holm, G. (1974). *Clin. Exp. Immunol.* **17**, 371.

Metzger, W. D., Miller, A., and Sercaz, E. (1980). *Fed. Proc., Fed. Am. Soc. Exp. Biol.* **39**, 572.

Miller, J. F. A. P., Vadas, M. A., Whitelaw, A., and Gamble, J. (1976). *Proc. Natl. Acad. Sci. U.S.A.* **73**, 2486.

Mitchison, N. A. (1980). *In* "Federal Symposium of Independent Society of Cell Biology" (K. B. Vernon, ed.), p. 5. Academic Press, New York.

Mitchison, N. A. (1971). *Eur. J. Immunol* 1, 18.

Mond, J. J., Lieberman, R., Inman, J. K., Mosier, D. E., and Paul, W. E. (1977). *J. Exp. Med.* 146, 1138.

Morse, H. C., III, Prescott, B., Cross, S. S., Stashak, P. W., and Baker, P. J. (1976). *J. Immunol.* 116, 279.

Mozes, E., and Haimovich, J. (1979). *Nature (London)* 278, 56.

Mudawwar, F. D., Yunis, E. J., and Geha, R. S. (1978). *J. Exp. Med.* 148, 1032.

Mudgett, M., Coligan, J. E. and Kindt, T. J. (1978). *J. Immunol.* 120, 293.

Munro, A., Tausig, M., Cambell, B., Williams, H., and Lawson, Y. (1974). *J. Exp. Med.* 140, 1579.

Mushinski, E. B., and Potter, M. (1977). *J. Immunol.* 119, 1888.

Nisonoff, A., Ju, S.-T. and Owen, F. L. (1977). *Immunol. Rev.* 34, 89.

Nutt, N. B. Wiesel, A. N., and Nisonoff, A. (1979). *Eur. J. Immunol.* 9, 864.

Osmond, D. G. (1979). *In* "B Lymphocytes in the Immune Response" (M. Cooper, D. E. Mosier, I. Scher, and E. S. Vitetta, eds.), Vol. 3, p. 63. Elsevier-North Holland, New York.

Oudin, J. (1980). *J. Exp. Med.* 112, 107.

Oudin, J., and Bordenave, G. (1971). *Nature (London)* 231, 86.

Oudin, J., and Cazenave, P. A. (1971). *Proc. Natl. Acad. Sci. U.S.A.* 68, 2616.

Oudin, J., and Michel, M. (1963). *C. R. Hebd. Seances. Acad. Sci.* 251, 805.

Oudin, J., and Michel, M. (1969a). *J. Exp. Med.* 130, 545.

Oudin, J., and Michel, M. (1969b). *J. Exp. Med.* 130, 619.

Owen, F. L., and Nisonoff, A. (1978). *J. Exp. Med.* 149, 182.

Owen, F. L., Ju, S.-T., and Nisonoff, A. (1979a). *J. Exp. Med.* 145, 1559.

Owen, F. L., Ju, S.-T., and Nisonoff, A. (1979b). *Proc. Natl. Acad. Sci. U.S.A.* 74, 2084.

Owen, F. L., Ju, S.-T., and Nisonoff, A. (1977). *Proc. Natl. Acad. Sci. U.S.A.* 74, 2084.

Owen, J. J. T. (1979). *In* "B Lymphocytes in the Immune Response" (M. Cooper, D. E. Mosier, I. Scher, and E. S. Vitetta, eds.), Vol. 3, p. 71. Elsevier-North Holland, New York.

Patrick, J., and Lindstrom, J. M. (1973). *Science* 180, 871.

Paul, W. E., Subbarao, B., Mond, J. J., Sieckmann, D. G., Zitron, I., Ahmed, A., Mosier, D. E., and Scher, I. (1979). *In* "Cells of Immunoglobulin Synthesis" (B. Pernis and H. Vogel, eds.), p. 383. Academic Press, New York.

Pawlak, L. L. Mushinski, E. B., Nisonoff, A., and Potter, M. (1973a). *J. Exp. Med.* 137, 22.

Pawlak, L. L., Hart, D. A., and Nisonoff, A. (1973b). *J. Exp. Med.* 137, 1442.

Penn, G., Kunkel, H., and Grey, H. (1970). *Proc. Soc. Exp. Biol. Med.* 135, 660.

Pernis, B., Chiappino, G., Kelus, A. S., and Gell, P. G. H. (1970). *J. Exp. Med.* 122, 853.

Pincus, S. H., Sachs, D. H., and Dickler, H. B. (1978). *J. Immunol.* 121, 1422.

Pisetsky, D. S., Riordan, S. E., and Sachs, D. H. (1979). *J. Immunol.* 122, 842.

Potter, M. (1977). *Advan. Immunol.* 25, 141.

Potter, M., and Boyce, C. R. (1962). *Nature (London)* 133, 1086.

Potter, M., Rudikoff, S., Vrana, M., Rao, D. N., and Mushinski, E. B. (1977). *Cold Spring Harbor Symp. Quant. Biol.* 41, 661.

Potter, M., Mushinski, E. B., Rudikoff, S., Glaudemans, C. P. J., Padlan, E. A., and Davies, D. R. (1979). *Ann. Immunol. (Paris)* 130C, 263.

Prahl, J. W., and Porter, R. R. (1968). G *Biochem. J.* 107, 753.

Prange, C. A., Fiedler, J., Nitecki, D. E., and Bellone, C. J. (1977). *J. Exp. Med.* 146, 766.

Preud'homme, J. L., Klein, M., Labaume, S., and Seligman, M. (1977). *Eur. J. Immunol.* 7, 840.

Raff, M. C., Sternberg, M., and Taylor, R. B. (1970). *Nature (London)* 225, 456.

Raff, M. C., Megson, M., Owen, J. J. T., and Cooper, M. D. (1976). *Nature (London)* 259, 224.

Ramasier, H. (1973). *Curr. Topics Microbiol. Immunol.* 60, 31.

Ramseier, H. (1975). *Eur. J. Immunol.* 5, 23.

Ramseier, H., and Lindemann, J. (1971). *J. Exp. Med.* 134, 1083.

Ramseier, H., and Lindemann, J. (1972). *Transplant. Rev.* 10, 57.

Rao, D. N., Rudikoff, S., and Potter, M. (1978). *Biochemistry* 17, 5555.

Ray, A., and Cebra, J. J. (1972). *Biochemistry* 11, 3647.

Reth, M., Hammerling, G. J., and Rajewsky, K. (1978). *Eur. J. Immunol.* 8, 383.

Riblet, R., Blomberg, B., Weigert, M., Lieberman, R., Taylor, B. A., and Potter, M. (1975). *Eur. J. Immunol.* 5, 775.

Richter, P. H. (1975). *Eur. J. Immunol.* 5, 350.

Riesen, W. F. (1979). *Eur. J. Immunol.* 9, 421.

Rodkey, L. S. (1974). *J. Exp. Med.* 139, 712.

Roland, J., and Cazenave, P. A. (1979). *C. R. Hebd. Seances. Acad. Sci.* 288, 571.

Rosenberg, Y. J., and Parish, C. R. (1977). *J. Immunol.* 118, 612.

Rowley, D. A., Miller, G. W., and Lorbach, I. (1978). *J. Exp. Med.* 148, 148.

Rozing, J., Brous, N. H. C., and Denner, R. (1977). *Cell. Immunol.* 29, 37.

Rubin, B., Hertel-Wulff, B., and Kimura, A. (1979). *J. Exp. Med.* 150, 307.

Rudikoff, S., and Potter, M. (1974). *Biochemistry* 13, 4033.

Saint Martin, J., Mukoyama, H., and Eyquem, A. (1978). *C. R. Hebd. Seances Acad. Sci.* 287, 1183.

Sakato, N., and Eisen, H. N. (1975). *J. Exp. Med.* 141, 1411.

Salsano, F., Froland, S. S., Natvig, J. B., and Michaelsen, T. E. (1974). *Scand. J. Immunol.* 3, 841.

Schiff, C., Boyer, C., Millili, M., and Fougereau, M. (1979). *Eur. J. Immunol.*

Schilling, J., Clevinger, B., Davie, J. M., and Hood, L. (1980). *Nature (London)* 283, 35.

Schimpl, A., and Wecker, E. (1972). *Nature (London), New Biol.* 237, 15.

Schrater, A. F., Goidl, A., Thorbecke, G. J., and Siskind, G. W. (1979a). *J. Exp. Med.* 150, 138.

Schrater, A. F., Goidl, A., Thorbecke, G. J., and Siskind, G. W. (1979b). *J. Exp. Med.* 150, 808.

Schroer, K. R., Briles, D. E., Van Boxel, J. A., and Davie, J. M. (1974). *J. Exp. Med.* 140, 1416.

Schroer, K. R., Kim, K. J., Amsbaugh, D. F., Stashak, P. W., and Baker, P. J. (personal communication).

Schuler, W., Weiler, E., and Kolb, H. (1977). *Eur. J. Immunol.* 7, 649.

Schwartz, M., Kifshitz, R., Givol, D., Mozes, E., and Haimovich, J. (1978a). *J. Immunol.* 121, 421.

Schwartz, M., Novick, D., Givol, D., and Fuchs, S. (1978b). *Nature (London)* 273, 543.

Sege, K., and Peterson, P. A. (1978a). *Nature (London)* 271, 157.

Sege, K., and Peterson, P. A. (1978b). *Proc. Natl. Acad. Sci. U.S.A.* 75, 2443.

Sell, S., and Gell, P. G. H. (1965). *J. Exp. Med.* **122**, 423.

Seppälä, I. G. T., and Eichmann, K. (1979). *Eur. J. Immunol.* **9**, 243.

Serban, D., Ran, M., and Witz, I. P. (1979). *Cell. Immunol.* **44**, 1.

Shearer, G. M., Rehn, T. G., and Schmitt-Vershulst, A. M. (1976) *Transplant. Rev.* **23**, 222.

Shen, F. W., McDougal, J. S., Bard, J., and Cort, S. P. (1980). *J. Exp. Med.* **151**, 566.

Sher, A., and Cohn, M. (1972). *J. Immunol.* **109**, 176.

Sherman, L. A., Burakoff, S. J., and Benacerraf, B. (1978). *J. Immunol.* **121**, 1432.

Sidman, C. L., and Unanue, E. R. (1978). *Proc. Natl. Acad. Sci. U.S.A.* **75**, 2401.

Sieckmann, D. G., Asofsky, R., Mosier, D. E., Zitron, I. M., and Paul, W. E. (1978). *J. Exp. Med.* **147**, 814.

Signal, N. H., Gearhart, P. J., Press, J. L., and Klinman, N. R. (1976). *Nature (London)* **253**, 51.

Silverstein, A. M. (1977). In "Development of Host Defense" (M. D. Cooper and D. H. Deyton, eds.) pp. 1–19. Raven, New York.

Silverstein, A. M., and Kramer, K. L. (1965). In "Molecular and Cellular basis of Antibody Formation" (J. Sterzl, ed.), p. 341. Academic Press, New York.

Singhal, S. K., Roder, J. C., and Duwe, A. K. (1978). *Fed. Proc., Fed. Am. Soc. Exp. Biol.* **37**, 1245.

Sirisinha, S., and Eisen, H. H. (1971). *Proc. Natl. Acad. Sci. U.S.A.* **68**, 3130.

Siskind, G. N. (1979). In "B Lymphocyte in the Immune Response" (M. D. Cooper, D. E. Mosier, I. Scher, and E. Vitetta, eds.), Vol. 3, p. 85. Elsevier-North Holland, New York.

Slater, R. J., Ward, S. M., and Kunkel, H. G. (1955). *J. Exp. Med.* **101**, 85.

Somme, G., Petit, C. and Th J. (1979).

Spear, P. P., and Edelman, G. M. (1974). *J. Exp. Med.* **139**, 249.

Spear, P. G., Wang, A., Rutishausen, U., and Edelman, G. M. (1973). *J. Exp. Med.* **138**, 557.

Stanislawski, M. (1981). In "Lymphocytic Regulation by Antibodies" (C. Bona and P. A. Cazenave, eds.), p. 21. Wiley, New York.

Stanley, E. F., and Drachman, D. B. (1978). *Science* **200**, 1285.

Stein, K. E., Bona, C., Lieberman, R., Chien, C. C., and Paul, W. E. (1980). *J. Exp. Med.* **151**, 1088.

Strayer, D. S., Lee, W. M. F., Rowley, D., and Kohler, H. (1975). *J. Immunol.* **114**, 728.

Streefkerk, D. G., Vrana, M., and Glandemaus, C. P. J. (1978). *J. Immunol.* **120**, 408.

Stuart, F. P., Scollard, D. M., McKearn, T. J., and Fitch, F. W. (1976). *Transplantation* **22**, 455.

Sugai, S., Palmer, D. P., Talal, N., and Witz, I. P. (1974). *J. Exp. Med.* **140**, 1547.

Sugiyama, H., Benda, P., Meunier, P., and Changeux, J. C. (1973). *FEBS Lett.* **35**, 124.

Sy, M. S., Bach, B. A., Dohi, Y., Nisonoff, A., Benacerraf, B., and Green, M. I., (1979a). *J. Exp. Med.* **150**, 1216.

Sy, M. A., Bach, B. A., Brown, A., Nisonoff, A., Benacerraf, B., and Green, M. I. (1979b). *J. Exp. Med.* **150**, 1223.

Sy, M. S., Moorhead, J. W., and Claman, H. N. (1979c). *J. Immunol.* **123**, 2593.

Sy, M. S., Brown, A. R., Benacerraf, B., and Green, M. I. (1980). *J. Exp. Med.* **151**, 896.

Tada, T., Taniguchi, M., and Okumura, K. (1978). *J. Supermolec. Struct. Suppl.* **3**, 236.

Tasiaux, N., Lewenkroon, R., Bruyus, C., and Urbain, J. (1978). *Eur. J. Immunol.* **8**, 464.

Trenkner, E., and Riblet, R. (1975). *J. Exp. Med.* 142, 1121.

Tzartos, S. J., and Lindstrom, J. M. (1980). *Proc. Natl. Acad. Sci. U.S.A.* 77, 755.

Urbain, J. (1977). *Ann. Immunol. (Paris)* 128C, 445.

Urbain, J., Wikler, M., Franssen, J. D., and Collignon, C. (1977). *Proc. Natl. Acad. Sci. U.S.A.* 74, 5126.

Vadas, M. A., Miller, J. F. A. P., Whitelaw, A. M., and Gamble, J. R. (1976). *Immunogenetics (N.Y.)* 4, 137.

Vitetta, E. S., Uhr. J. W., and Boyse, E. A. (1973). *Proc. Natl. Acad. Sci. U.S.A.* 70, 834.

Vrana, M., Rudikoff, S., and Potter, M. (1978). *Proc. Natl. Acad. Sci. U.S.A.* 75, 1957.

Wang, A. C., Wilson, S. K., Hopper, J. E., Fudenberg, H. H., and Nisonoff, A. (1970). *Proc. Natl. Acad. Sci. U.S.A.* 66, 337.

Ward, K., Cantor, H., and Boyse, E. A. (1978a). *In* "The Immune System: Genetics and Regulation" (E. S. Sercaz, L. A. Herzenberg, and C. F. Fox, eds.), p. 397. Academic Press, New York.

Ward, K., Cantor, H., and Nisonoff, A. (1978b). *J. Immunol.* 120, 2016.

Weigert, M., and Riblet, R. (1978). *Springer Semin. Immunopathol.* 1, 133.

Weigert, M., Reschke, W. C., Carson, D., and Cohn, M. (1974). *J. Exp. Med.* 139, 137.

Weigle, O. W., and Parks, D. E. (1978). *Fed. Proc., Fed. Am. Soc. Exp. Biol.* 37, 1253.

Weigle, O. W., and Berman, A. M. (1979). *In* "Cells of Immunoglobulin Synthesis" (B. Pernis and H. J. Vogel, eds.), p. 223. Academic Press, New York.

Weiler, I. J. (1981) *In* "Lymphocytic Regulation by Antibodies" (C. Bona and P. A. Cazenave, eds.), p. 245. Wiley, New York.

Weiler, I. J., Weiler, E., Sprenger, R., and Cosenza, H. (1977). *Eur. J. Immunol.* 7, 531.

Weinberg, C. B., and Hall, Z. W. (1979). *Proc. Natl. Acad. Sci. U.S.A.* 76, 504.

Weinberger, J. Z., Germain, R. N., Ju, S.-T., Green, M. I., Benacerraf, B., and Dorf, M. E. (1979). *J. Exp. Med.* 150, 761.

Wells, J. V. (1973). *Proc. Natl. Acad. Sci. U.S.A.* 70, 1585.

Wells, J. V. H., Fudenberg, H., and Givol, D. (1973). *Proc. Natl. Acad. Sci. U.S.A.* 70, 1585.

Wernet, P., Feizi, T., and Kunkel, H. G. (1972). *J. Exp. Med.* 138, 965.

Wikler, M. Franssen, J. D., Collignon, C., Leo, O., Mariame, B., van de Walle, P., de Groote, D., and Urbain, J. (1979). *J. Exp. Med.* 150, 184.

Williams, R. C., Kunkel, H. G., and Capra, J. D. (1968). *Science* 161, 379.

Wilson, D. B., Smilek, D., and Bellgrau, D. (1980). *In* "Regulatory T Lymphocytes" (B. Pernis and H. Vogel, eds.), p. 15. Academic Press, New York.

Yamada, A., Adler, L. T., and Adler, F. L. (1979). *J. Exp. Med.* 150, 888.

Yamamoto, H., Nonaka, M., and Katz, D. (1979). *J. Exp. Med.* 150, 818.

Zanetti, M., and Bigazzi, P. E. (1980). *Fed. Proc., Fed. Am. Soc. Exp. Biol.* 39, 456.

Zeldis, J. B., Riblet, R., Konigsberg, W. H., Richards, F. L., and Rosenstein, R. W. (1979). *Mol. Immunol.* 26, 657.

Index

A

Accessory cell, 52-53, 157
Acetylcholine receptor, 184, 185, 189-190
Activation
  antibody-forming cells, 82-83
  B cells, 83, 97, 105, 136
  clone, 74
  T cells, 130
  V gene, 45-58
Addison's disease, 183
Agglutination, inhibition by antibody, 7
Alloantibody, 107
Alloantigen, 78, 106, 117, 118, 121, 152, 155, 170
Allograft, see Graft resistance; Graft versus host reaction
Allotype, 157, 170
  dominance, 99
  $Ig-1^a$, 145-147
  Lewis, 116-117
  linkage to $Igh-C$ gene, 6, 26
  specificity, 26
  suppression, 62, 85-86, 102
Anemia, pernicious, 184
Antibody, see also Alloantibody; Autoantibody

anti-allotypic, 6-8, 9, 19, 40, 85
anti-idiotypic, 3, 5, 8-12, 22, 23, 44, 62, 66, 83, 87-88, 89, 91, 102-104, 107, 165-166
  activation of antibody-forming cells, 82-83
  antigen mimicry, 163, 165, 166
  complementary, 160-163
  hypersensivity effect, 123-126
  in autoimmune disease, 191-192
  network theory, 157-159
  regulation of lymphocyte function, 156-182
  silent clone stimulation, 178-182
  spontaneous occurrence, 70-75, 182
  T cell proliferative response effect, 121-123, 151-155
anti-receptor, 183-186
auto, see Autoantibody
autoanti-receptor, 182
diversity, 6, 44, 58, 106, 158
evolution, 13, 23, 25, 57-58
heterogeneity, 36
immunogenicity, 2
maternal production, 44
monoclonal, 7, 8-9, 22-23, 51, 69
nonlymphoid somatic cell modulation, 183-186

205

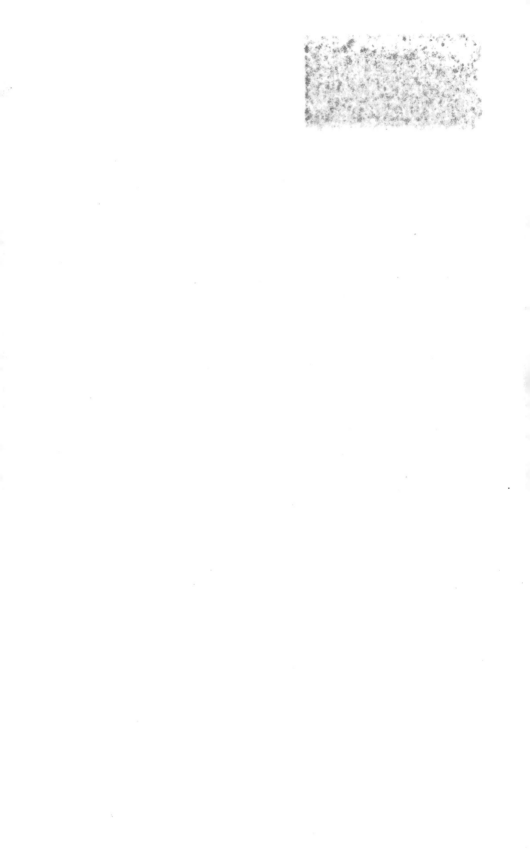